WORKBOOK TO ACCOMPANY

Introduction to Health Care

© 2017 Cengage Learning. All Rights Reserved. May not be scanned, copied or duplicated, or posted to a publicly accessible website, in whole or in part.

WORKBOOK TO ACCOMPANY

Introduction to Health Care

FOURTH EDITION

Dakota Mitchell, RN, MSN, MBA

Lee Haroun, EdD, MBA, MA Education

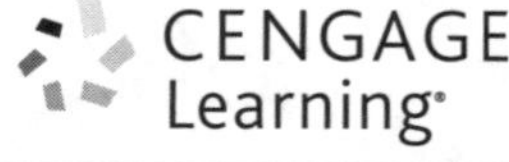

Australia • Brazil • Mexico • Singapore • United Kingdom • United States

© 2017 Cengage Learning. All Rights Reserved. May not be scanned, copied or duplicated, or posted to a publicly accessible website, in whole or in part.

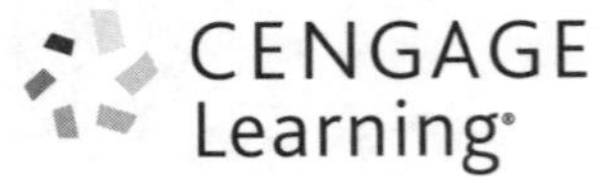

Workbook to Accompany Introduction to Health Care, Fourth Edition
Dakota Mitchell and Lee Haroun

SVP, GM Skills & Global Product Management: Dawn Gerrain

Product Director: Matthew Seeley

Senior Director, Development: Marah Bellegarde

Senior Product Development Manager: Juliet Steiner

Product Manager: Laura Stewart

Senior Content Developer: Debra M. Myette-Flis

Product Assistant: Deborah Handy

Vice President, Marketing Services: Jennifer Ann Baker

Marketing Manager: Cassie Cloutier

Marketing Coordinator: Courtney Cozzy

Senior Production Director: Wendy Troeger

Production Director: Andrew Crouth

Senior Content Project Manager: Kenneth McGrath

Managing Art Director: Jack Pendleton

Cover image(s): © iStock.com/zokara, © iStock.com/jonya, © iStock.com/svetkid, © iStock.com/Christopher Futcher, © iStock.com/sudok1, © Shutterstock/Tyler Olsen, © Shutterstock/Bullstar

© 2017, 2012 Cengage Learning

ALL RIGHTS RESERVED. No part of this work covered by the copyright herein may be reproduced or distributed in any form or by any means, except as permitted by U.S. copyright law, without the prior written permission of the copyright owner.

For product information and technology assistance, contact us at
Cengage Learning Customer & Sales Support, 1-800-354-9706
For permission to use material from this text or product,
submit all requests online at **www.cengage.com/permissions.**
Further permissions questions can be e-mailed to
permissionrequest@cengage.com

Library of Congress Control Number: 2015955717

ISBN: 978-1-3055-7495-3

Cengage Learning
20 Channel Center Street
Boston, MA 02210
USA

Cengage Learning is a leading provider of customized learning solutions with employees residing in nearly 40 different countries and sales in more than 125 countries around the world. Find your local representative at **www.cengage.com.**

Cengage Learning products are represented in Canada by Nelson Education, Ltd.

To learn more about Cengage Learning, visit **www.cengage.com**
Purchase any of our products at your local college store or at our preferred online store **www.cengagebrain.com**

Notice to the Reader
Publisher does not warrant or guarantee any of the products described herein or perform any independent analysis in connection with any of the product information contained herein. Publisher does not assume, and expressly disclaims, any obligation to obtain and include information other than that provided to it by the manufacturer. The reader is expressly warned to consider and adopt all safety precautions that might be indicated by the activities described herein and to avoid all potential hazards. By following the instructions contained herein, the reader willingly assumes all risks in connection with such instructions. The publisher makes no representations or warranties of any kind, including but not limited to, the warranties of fitness for particular purpose or merchantability, nor are any such representations implied with respect to the material set forth herein, and the publisher takes no responsibility with respect to such material. The publisher shall not be liable for any special, consequential, or exemplary damages resulting, in whole or part, from the readers' use of, or reliance upon, this material.

Printed in the United States of America
Print Number: 01 Print Year: 2015

© 2017 Cengage Learning. All Rights Reserved. May not be scanned, copied or duplicated, or posted to a publicly accessible website, in whole or in part.

Table of Contents

© 2017 Cengage Learning. All Rights Reserved. May not be scanned, copied or duplicated, or posted to a publicly accessible website, in whole or in part.

UNIT 6 Communication in the Health Care Setting 127

UNIT 7 Health Care Skills 165

UNIT 8 Business of Caring 185

UNIT 9 Securing and Maintaining Employment 203

© 2017 Cengage Learning. All Rights Reserved. May not be scanned, copied or duplicated, or posted to a publicly accessible website, in whole or in part.

To the Learner

Introduction to Health Care, fourth edition, is designed as an introductory text for learners who are entering college-level health care programs or for those who believe they may be interested in pursuing a career in health care. The fundamentals common to all health care occupations are presented in this full-color text to create a foundation on which learners can build when they take their specific occupational courses. The topics included are appropriate for occupations that involve direct patient care, such as nursing and dental assisting, as well as those that provide support services, such as health information technology and pharmacy technician. The goal of the text is to present a broad base of health care essentials. Therefore, skills and procedures that apply only to specific occupations are not included.

ORGANIZATION OF THE WORKBOOK

The purpose of this workbook is to provide you with additional practice to help you master content in the textbook. Each chapter in the workbook corresponds to the same chapter in the textbook and begins with the statement of chapter objectives. A variety of questions and exercises are included to help reinforce in different ways the material you have learned. Types of questions and exercises included in the workbook include defining terms, matching, identification, true/false, true/false rewrite, multiple choice, completion, ordering, and labeling. Additionally, each chapter includes two critical thinking scenarios to encourage you to think about and apply concepts learned in the chapter. Procedure checklists are also included to help you assess your mastery of the basic hands-on skills included in the text.

As you proceed through each chapter of the text, complete the activities provided in this workbook to reinforce the material presented in class.

The following steps are recommended for using the textbook and workbook:

1. Read the chapter objectives.
2. Study the material presented in the text.
3. Listen carefully to the instructor.
4. Take comprehensive notes.
5. Ask questions.
6. Complete the questions and exercises in the workbook.
7. Review any concepts missed while completing the workbook exercises.

This workbook was prepared as a tool to help you learn. The authors hope this tool will help you master the introductory health care concepts necessary for success in your chosen career.

© 2017 Cengage Learning. All Rights Reserved. May not be scanned, copied or duplicated, or posted to a publicly accessible website, in whole or in part.

UNIT 1
Health Care Today

© 2017 Cengage Learning. All Rights Reserved. May not be scanned, copied or duplicated, or posted to a publicly accessible website, in whole or in part.

CHAPTER 1

Your Career in Health Care

LEARNING OBJECTIVES

Studying and applying the material in this chapter will help you to:

- Understand the state of the health care industry, including employment projections.
- Describe the essential core qualities demonstrated by effective health care professionals.
- Describe the major kinds of approvals whose purpose is to ensure the competency of health care professionals.
- List the personal factors that should be considered when choosing a health care career.
- Describe the four classifications of health care careers and give examples of three occupational titles for each classification.
- State the educational and certification, registration, and/or licensing requirements of occupations in which you are interested.
- Explain the meaning of "learning for mastery."
- Use study techniques that complement your preferred learning style.
- Practice the habits that contribute to both academic and professional success.
- Describe the advantages and challenges experienced by adult learners.
- List techniques that adult learners can use to develop their personal organization and time management skills.
- Explain the meaning of "thinking like a health care professional."
- Apply the five-step problem-solving process to make effective decisions.

© 2017 Cengage Learning. All Rights Reserved. May not be scanned, copied or duplicated, or posted to a publicly accessible website, in whole or in part.

VOCABULARY REVIEW

Definitions

Write the definition of each of the following words or terms.

1. bias

____
____
____

2. integrity

____
____
____

3. learning style

____
____
____

4. manual dexterity

____
____
____

5. reliable

____
____
____

Matching 1

Match the following terms with their correct definitions.

____	1. career ladder	A.	process of determining whether an individual has met predetermined standards
____	2. certification	B.	granting of permission to legally perform certain acts
____	3. licensure	C.	skills that practitioners of a specific occupation may legally perform
____	4. registration	D.	levels within an occupational area that require different amounts of education and training
____	5. scope of practice	E.	placement on an official list after meeting educational and testing requirements

© 2017 Cengage Learning. All Rights Reserved. May not be scanned, copied or duplicated, or posted to a publicly accessible website, in whole or in part.

Matching 2

Match the following terms with their correct definitions.

____ 1.	assessment	A.	belief not necessarily based on facts
____ 2.	objective data	B.	information that cannot be observed or measured
____ 3.	opinion	C.	factual approach to a situation
____ 4.	problem-solving process	D.	factors, such as a fever, that are observable or measurable
____ 5.	signs	E.	indication of disease or injury experienced by a patient
____ 6.	subjective data	F.	gathering of information to help determine a patient's condition
____ 7.	symptom	G.	sequence of steps used to help find solutions

Word Fill

Complete the following sentences by filling in the missing words.

diagnostic therapeutic kinesthetic visual
auditory

1. Nursing is an example of a/an ______________ occupation.
2. Radiologic technologist is an example of a/an ______________ occupation.
3. A good method for a/an ______________ learner to acquire new anatomical terms is by studying illustrations of the body systems.
4. Reading a list of medical terms aloud is a good way for a/an ______________ learner to master new vocabulary.
5. A/an ______________ learner would likely benefit by assembling a kit of the skeleton to learn the names of the bones.

CHAPTER REVIEW

Identification

Place an "X" in front of each therapeutic occupation.

____ 1. dental hygienist

____ 2. diagnostic medical sonographer

____ 3. pharmacy technician

____ 4. home health aide

____ 5. dietetic technician

____ 6. mental health technician

____ 7. medical transcriptionist

© 2017 Cengage Learning. All Rights Reserved. May not be scanned, copied or duplicated, or posted to a publicly accessible website, in whole or in part.

_____ 8. medical laboratory technician

_____ 9. medical assistant

_____ 10. paramedic

True/False

Indicate whether the following statements are true (T) or false (F).

_____ 1. Some health care occupations have more than one form of approval or certification.

_____ 2. Many adult learners are at a disadvantage when they try to compete with younger learners.

_____ 3. Some certifying and licensing boards require that test applicants graduate from an accredited program.

_____ 4. Manual dexterity refers to an individual's ability to observe.

_____ 5. The majority of learning involves memorizing facts, such as medical terms and the steps for performing procedures.

_____ 6. Individuals who have been convicted of specific crimes cannot take the certification exams for certain health care occupations.

_____ 7. Some health care employers require background checks and drug testing of job applicants.

_____ 8. Learning for mastery means studying the information required to pass tests.

_____ 9. Good instructors spend most class time telling learners only what they need to know to pass their exams.

_____ 10. Understanding why something is done in health care is as important as knowing how to do it.

Multiple Choice

Circle the best answer for each of the following questions. There is only one correct answer to each question.

1. The first step in the five-step problem-solving process is to _______________.

   A. gather information needed to solve the problem
   B. identify the real problem
   C. decide if the problem is worth trying to solve

2. What is the last step when using the five-step problem-solving process?

   A. take action by implementing a solution
   B. review the results of the action taken
   C. choose an alternative

© 2017 Cengage Learning. All Rights Reserved. May not be scanned, copied or duplicated, or posted to a publicly accessible website, in whole or in part.

3. Which of the following individuals best demonstrates the meaning of "thinking like a health care professional"?

   A. Dan, a surgical technologist, has learned a series of steps that he always uses when preparing a patient for surgery.
   B. Angie, a laboratory technician, always collects the materials she will need before performing lab tests.
   C. Jacob, a veterinary technician, brings to the veterinarian's attention unusual behavior in a dog that was brought in for a test.

4. Which of the following challenges is most likely to be faced by an adult returning to school?

   A. finding time to study
   B. competing with younger students
   C. lack of self-confidence

5. Which of the following activities would most likely work best for a visual learner who is studying the characteristics of good medical documentation?

   A. read about each of the characteristics
   B. practice creating samples of medical documentation
   C. say the characteristics out loud

6. Brandon is interested in the field of physical therapy, but does not currently have a lot of time or the financial resources to attend school. Which of the following physical therapy careers would be best under these circumstances?

   A. physical therapist
   B. physical therapist aide
   C. physical therapist assistant

7. Which of the following careers would best suit an individual who enjoys working with detailed paperwork?

   A. optometric assistant
   B. magnetic resonance technologist
   C. coding specialist

8. Which of the following certifications is never voluntary?

   A. licensure
   B. certification
   C. approval

9. Jeff enjoys the lecture portion of his *Introduction to Health Care* class, but dislikes any kind of group work with his classmates. How is this likely to affect his future career success?

   A. no effect as long as he performs his work
   B. positively because he will not waste his time socializing with coworkers
   C. negatively because work in health care is performed by teams

10. Which of the following individuals is expressing an opinion?

    A. Mike: "People who don't have jobs and lack medical insurance are just too lazy to work."
    B. James: According to the Bureau of Labor Statistics, the unemployment rate in the United States is 9.5%."
    C. Dan: "The best way to help the homeless is by volunteering at a local community center."

© 2017 Cengage Learning. All Rights Reserved. May not be scanned, copied or duplicated, or posted to a publicly accessible website, in whole or in part.

Matching 3

Match the following core qualities of health care professionals with the example that best demonstrates that quality.

_____ 1. care about others	A.	use courtesy with coworkers
_____ 2. have integrity	B.	never take supplies for your own use
_____ 3. be dependable	C.	accept responsibility for an error made at work
_____ 4. work well with others	D.	read articles that relate to your career area
_____ 5. be flexible	E.	return from lunch break on schedule
_____ 6. be willing to learn	F.	show respect to a difficult patient
_____ 7. strive to be cost conscious	G.	exchange work days to help at a weekend flu clinic

Completion

Use the words in the list to complete the following statements.

technologist	license	assistant	registration
associate's	certification	bachelor's	standards
scope of practice	aide		

1. _______________ for health care professionals are set by various agencies and organizations to ensure the professionals are competent.
2. _______________ means being placed on an official list after meeting certain educational and testing requirements.
3. The general term for describing the process of determining the competence of a health care professional is _______________.
4. An individual who is legally approved to work in a specific occupation receives a/an _______________.
5. The list of duties that can be performed by practitioners of a specific occupation is called its _______________.
6. The health care professional who has less education than an occupational therapy assistant is an occupational therapy _______________.
7. A physical therapist has more education than a physical therapist _______________.
8. A/An _______________ degree is usually completed in two years
9. A/An _______________ degree is usually completed in four years.
10. In most occupational areas, a/an _______________ has more education than a technician.

© 2017 Cengage Learning. All Rights Reserved. May not be scanned, copied or duplicated, or posted to a publicly accessible website, in whole or in part.

Ordering

Place the following positions on the emergency medical career ladder in the order of education required. Put a numeral 1 before the position requiring the most education, a 2 before the next, and so on.

_____ first responder

_____ EMT—Intermediate/99

_____ paramedic

_____ EMT—Basic

_____ EMT—Intermediate/85

Critical Thinking Scenarios

Read each scenario. Think about the information presented in the text, and then answer each question.

1. Craig finds it difficult to master new material unless he actually does something with it. For example, when learning a new procedure, it is hard for him to simply visualize the steps to follow.

   A. What type of learner is Craig?

   ____

   ____

   ____

   B. What study techniques can he use to best learn new information, such as the steps in the problem-solving process?

   ____

   ____

   ____

2. Mr. Taylor, a patient recovering from knee replacement surgery, tells Carla, a physical therapist assistant, that he is experiencing pain as he performs the exercises prescribed for him.

   A. Is the pain he is experiencing a sign or a symptom?

   ____

   ____

   ____

© 2017 Cengage Learning. All Rights Reserved. May not be scanned, copied or duplicated, or posted to a publicly accessible website, in whole or in part.

B. What is the difference between a sign and a symptom?

C. Is his pain an example of objective or subjective data?

© 2017 Cengage Learning. All Rights Reserved. May not be scanned, copied or duplicated, or posted to a publicly accessible website, in whole or in part.

CHAPTER 2

Current Health Care Systems and Trends

LEARNING OBJECTIVES

Studying and applying the material in this chapter will help you to:

- Describe 10 significant events in the history of health care that changed the way care was delivered.
- Describe the major forces in the health care industry today.
- Describe the levels of care offered by the modern hospital.
- List 10 ambulatory health care facilities and give examples of the type of services offered by each one.
- Describe the major types of long-term care facilities.
- Provide examples of health care services and care that can be provided in the patient's home.
- Explain the purpose of hospice.
- List typical services offered by federal, state, and local health agencies.
- Explain the concept of wellness.
- Describe the types of complementary and alternative medicine being practiced in the United States today.
- List five challenges facing health care today and explain how the health care professional can contribute to their resolution.

© 2017 Cengage Learning. All Rights Reserved. May not be scanned, copied or duplicated, or posted to a publicly accessible website, in whole or in part.

VOCABULARY REVIEW

Definitions

Write the definition of each of the following words or terms.

1. gene therapy

2. palliative

3. pandemic

4. psychosomatic

5. targeted drug therapy

6. vital statistics

7. dementia

8. opioids

© 2017 Cengage Learning. All Rights Reserved. May not be scanned, copied or duplicated, or posted to a publicly accessible website, in whole or in part.

Matching 1

Match the following terms with their correct definitions.

_____	1. acupuncture	A.	nontraditional treatment used along with conventional medicine
_____	2. alternative medicine	B.	combination of treatments from conventional medicine with complementary and/or alternative medicine
_____	3. chiropractic	C.	treatment involving insertion of tiny needles into the body
_____	4. complementary medicine	D.	treatment involving manipulating the spine to relieve pressure on nerves
_____	5. holistic medicine	E.	health care approach that considers all the following components: physical, mental, emotional, and spiritual
_____	6. integrative medicine	F.	medical theory that the body protects itself when the musculoskeletal system is in good order
_____	7. massage therapy	G.	treatment in which muscles are rubbed and kneaded
_____	8. osteopathy	H.	nontraditional treatment used instead of conventional medicine

Word Fill

Complete the following sentences by filling in the missing words.

intermediate nursing care facility	continuing care community	psychiatric	adult foster home
inpatient	assisted living residence	skilled nursing facility	outpatient
hospice	nursing home		

1. A/an ______________ provides personal care, meals, and supervision in a homelike setting for up to five or six residents.
2. A large live-in facility that provides housing, meals, and personal care is called a/an ______________.
3. A/an ______________ provides services at one location that range from independent living to nursing home care.
4. ______________ is a service or facility that provides care and support for individuals who are dying.
5. ______________ refers to being admitted to and treated in a hospital.
6. A nursing home that provides personal care, but not on a 24-hour basis, is called a/an ______________.
7. A/an ______________ is the general term for a live-in facility that provides nursing and personal care.

© 2017 Cengage Learning. All Rights Reserved. May not be scanned, copied or duplicated, or posted to a publicly accessible website, in whole or in part.

8. Medical services provided to patients who are not admitted to a hospital are called ______________ services.
9. In a/an ______________ hospital, patients are treated for mental and behavioral disorders.
10. A nursing home that provides 24-hour nursing care, along with personal care, is called a/an ______________.

CHAPTER REVIEW

True/False

Indicate whether the following statements are true (T) or false (F).

_____ 1. The typical lifespan in ancient times was only 45 years.

_____ 2. The Greek physician Hippocrates of Cos has been called the Father of Medicine.

_____ 3. The plagues of the Middle Ages killed more than half the population of Europe.

_____ 4. In the 17th century, William Harvey proposed the first theory of contagious diseases.

_____ 5. The microscope was invented in the mid 1800s.

_____ 6. The discovery that quinine treated malaria confirmed the theory that specific diseases have specific cures.

_____ 7. For many centuries, it was believed that mucous from a head cold was produced by the brain.

_____ 8. At one time, when diseases were not well understood, 2400 different diseases were “identified” because of slight differences in symptoms.

_____ 9. Before the mid-1700s, mental illness was not recognized as a disease, but thought to be the result of being possessed by the devil.

_____ 10. Edward Jenner demonstrated that vaccinations could be an effective preventive technique for smallpox.

_____ 11. Anesthesia was introduced by surgeons in the early 1900s.

_____ 12. Louis Pasteur developed the germ theory by proving that specific bacteria caused specific diseases.

_____ 13. The theory of psychoanalysis to treat mental illness was developed by Sigmund Freud.

_____ 14. Large-scale vaccination programs were started in the mid-1800s.

_____ 15. The influenza pandemic of 1918 killed about 2,000,000 people.

_____ 16. Vitamins and their effect on the human body were discovered in the 20th century.

_____ 17. In the 20th century, the scientific approach became the principal basis for the practice of medicine.

_____ 18. AIDS was identified as a disease in the 1960s.

_____ 19. Widespread media, such as the Internet, have decreased the spread of fraudulent quick-curing health products.

_____ 20. The first “test tube” baby was born in 1978.

© 2017 Cengage Learning. All Rights Reserved. May not be scanned, copied or duplicated, or posted to a publicly accessible website, in whole or in part.

True/False Rewrite

Please rewrite the bold part of the sentence to make the statement true.

1. Home care is **limited to basic services** such as nursing and assistance with personal care.

___

___

___

2. Medicare covers **all the costs** of home health services.

___

___

___

3. Home health agencies are generally **not regulated.**

___

___

___

4. Occupational therapists help patients **regain movement and increase their physical stamina.**

___

___

___

5. The National Institutes of Health **provide treatment for** chronic diseases such as cancer.

___

___

___

6. **Local health departments** license health care personnel and facilities.

___

___

___

7. The Occupational Safety and Health Administration **ensures that drugs are pure, safe, and effective.**

___

___

___

8. The Centers for Disease Control and Prevention is **supported by private financial donations.**

___

___

___

© 2017 Cengage Learning. All Rights Reserved. May not be scanned, copied or duplicated, or posted to a publicly accessible website, in whole or in part.

9. **Children and adolescents** are the heaviest users of health care services.

____

____

____

10. Many newly developed antibiotics are effective against **most viruses.**

____

____

____

Matching 2

Match the following facilities with the service offered in each.

_____	1. adult day care facility	A.	treatment and care for cancer or other specific condition
_____	2. dental office	B.	treatment for conditions that need immediate attention
_____	3. diagnostic center	C.	classes on nutrition and exercise
_____	4. urgent care center	D.	diagnosis and treatment of various health conditions
_____	5. laboratory	E.	activities, meals, and supervision for older and disabled individuals
_____	6. medical mall	F.	tests such as X-ray and ultrasound
_____	7. medical office	G.	physical and occupational therapy
_____	8. rehabilitation center	H.	operations, such as tonsil removal
_____	9. specialty clinic	I.	tests on blood and other body fluids
_____	10. surgical center	J.	care of the teeth
_____	11. wellness center	K.	a large variety of medical and health care services in one location

Short Answer

Read each question. Think about the information presented in the text, and then answer each question.

1. What are the factors influencing the rapid growth of home health services?

____

____

____

2. What is the currently held meaning of wellness? Include an explanation of the concept of "expanding consciousness."

____

____

____

© 2017 Cengage Learning. All Rights Reserved. May not be scanned, copied or duplicated, or posted to a publicly accessible website, in whole or in part.

3. Briefly discuss the following five challenges facing the health care community today.

   A. Providing long-term care for the elderly and disabled

   B. Providing care for patients with Alzheimer's disease

   C. Encouraging medication adherence

   D. Preventing prescription medication abuse

   E. Preventing antibiotic resistance

4. List at least five reasons for the increasing cost of health care.

5. What are three results of specialization in medicine and health care?

6. What are six categories of waste that contribute to the high cost of health care in the United States?

© 2017 Cengage Learning. All Rights Reserved. May not be scanned, copied or duplicated, or posted to a publicly accessible website, in whole or in part.

7. Compare and contrast the following types of medicine: alternative, complementary, and integrative.

____

____

____

8. Which segments of the population still struggle to pay for health care despite the passage of the Affordable Care Act?

____

____

____

Completion

Use the words in the list to complete the following statements:

traditional Chinese medicine	reiki	reflexology	acupuncture
aromatherapy	homeopathy	meditation	naturopathy
chiropractic	guided imagery	ayurveda	

1. ______________ is an ancient Chinese medicine treatment that uses needles to reduce pain.
2. The use of the hands to manipulate the spine to relieve pressure on the nerves is called ______________.
3. The medical system in which symptom-producing substances are administered based on the theory that "like cures like" is ______________.
4. ______________ is the theory of medicine that draws on nature and emphasizes treating the causes rather than just the symptoms of diseases and disorders.
5. ______________ is based on balancing and maintaining the body's energy flow.
6. Treatment that involves inhaling the scents of plant oils is called ______________.
7. The practice of ______________ by individuals has been found to help them integrate their physical and mental aspects.
8. ______________ is a 5000-year-old system of medicine practiced in India.
9. ______________ is based on the theory that parts of the bottom of the feet correspond to specific parts of the body.
10. Practitioners of ______________ use their hands in an effort to transmit healing energy to the body.
11. Words and music are used in ______________ to evoke positive mental scenes.

© 2017 Cengage Learning. All Rights Reserved. May not be scanned, copied or duplicated, or posted to a publicly accessible website, in whole or in part.

Ordering

Place the following levels of care offered in a hospital in order from the highest to the lowest.

_____ general unit

_____ trauma center

_____ intensive care unit

_____ transitional care unit

_____ emergency department

Critical Thinking Scenarios

Read each scenario. Think about the information presented in the text, and then answer each question.

1. James is a recent graduate who just passed the NCLEX-RN examination. He is excited about beginning his nursing career and looks forward to making a difference in the lives of his patients.

   A. Why will James be most likely to work with many elderly patients during his career?

   ____

   ____

   ____

   B. Discuss three challenges he will face working in the health care field.

   ____

   ____

   ____

   C. What types of health care facilities will offer the most employment opportunities for James?

   ____

   ____

   ____

2. Erin is beginning her career as an occupational therapy assistant in a rehabilitation hospital. She would like to set a good example for her patients.

   A. What are five behaviors that contribute to good health?

   ____

   ____

   ____

   B. What are the three leading causes of death in the United States that can in some cases be prevented by good health habits?

   ____

   ____

   ____

© 2017 Cengage Learning. All Rights Reserved. May not be scanned, copied or duplicated, or posted to a publicly accessible website, in whole or in part.

CHAPTER 3

Ethical and Legal Responsibilities

LEARNING OBJECTIVES

Studying and applying the material in this chapter will help you to:

- Explain the meaning of ethics and its importance in the practice of health care.
- State the purpose of professional codes of ethics.
- Explain the meaning of values and how they influence personal and professional behavior.
- Describe the relationship between ethics and law.
- List the eight major ethical principles that apply to health care and give examples of the laws that support each.
- Explain how each of the following presents ethical challenges to the health care community: euthanasia, organ transplants, and rationing of care.
- Explain the importance of patient consent and the possible consequences when actions are taken without the patient's consent.
- Give the definitions of express and implied consent.
- Describe the two major forms of advance directives.
- List the signs of child and elder abuse and state the actions that health care professionals should take in cases of suspected abuse.
- Explain the purpose of the federal schedule of controlled substances.
- Describe the importance of patient confidentiality and possible legal consequences when it is breached.
- Give examples of how the health care professional applies ethics on the job.

© 2017 Cengage Learning. All Rights Reserved. May not be scanned, copied or duplicated, or posted to a publicly accessible website, in whole or in part.

VOCABULARY REVIEW

Definitions

Write the definition of each of the following legal words or terms.

1. adult (legal)

____

____

____

2. agent

____

____

____

3. damages

____

____

____

4. emancipated minor

____

____

____

5. euthanasia

____

____

____

6. invasive procedure

____

____

____

7. mercy killing

____

____

____

8. respondeat superior

____

____

____

© 2017 Cengage Learning. All Rights Reserved. May not be scanned, copied or duplicated, or posted to a publicly accessible website, in whole or in part.

Matching 1

Match the following terms with their correct definitions.

_____	1. advance directive	A.	agreement reached after the parties have discussed specific terms and conditions
_____	2. consent	B.	legal document in which individuals appoint specific person(s) to act on their behalf if they become unable to make health care decisions for themselves
_____	3. contract	C.	actions of the parties form an unwritten agreement
_____	4. designation of health care surrogate	D.	general term for permission given
_____	5. express consent	E.	written documents that explain a patient's wishes regarding health care
_____	6. express contract	F.	part of an advance directive that outlines the type and extent of medical care to be given
_____	7. implied consent	G.	formal promise that is enforceable by law
_____	8. implied contract	H.	permission given by actions, such as making an appointment with a physician
_____	9. informed consent	I.	permission for a procedure to be performed after it and any possible consequences have been explained
_____	10. living will	J.	permission given in writing

Matching 2

Match the following terms with their correct definitions.

_____	1. autonomy	A.	intended to be kept secret; right to privacy
_____	2. code of ethics	B.	system of principles used to determine right and wrong
_____	3. confidentiality	C.	laws
_____	4. discreet	D.	beliefs about what is important that provide a foundation for making decisions
_____	5. ethical dilemma	E.	fundamental truths
_____	6. ethics	F.	taking care with what is said and respecting privacy
_____	7. justice	G.	self-determination
_____	8. legislation	H.	standard methods for performing tasks and procedures
_____	9. principles	I.	fairness
_____	10. protocols	J.	situation in which contradicting ethical principles collide
_____	11. values	K.	collection of principles to guide right conduct

© 2017 Cengage Learning. All Rights Reserved. May not be scanned, copied or duplicated, or posted to a publicly accessible website, in whole or in part.

Word Fill

Complete the following sentences by filling in the missing words.

negligence	libel	defamation of character	slander
breach of contract	assault	false imprisonment	battery
malpractice	fraud		

1. A nurse threatening a child with a spanking is an example of ________________.
2. If a patient states he does not want a treatment and the physician performs it anyway, the physician may be charged with ________________.
3. A patient who refuses to pay his dental bill for a crown he agreed to have made is committing a/an ________________.
4. ________________ is a legal charge for disclosing unauthorized information that could harm the reputation of another person.
5. A mentally competent patient who is hospitalized against his wishes may charge the hospital with ________________.
6. Making claims that an unproven method of treatment will cure cancer is an example of ________________.
7. Making a written statement that might harm a person's reputation may result in a charge of ________________.
8. A postsurgical patient who suffers an injury when his physical therapist recommends an obviously inappropriate exercise may decide to sue the therapist for ________________.
9. ________________ means the failure to provide the standard of care expected of a professional with specific training and experience.
10. Making false, harmful statements about someone whose reputation is then hurt might result in a charge of ________________.

CHAPTER REVIEW

True/False

Indicate whether the following statements are true (T) or false (F).

_____ 1. It is correct for a medical assistant to inform a patient if she believes the physician has not approved the most effective medication for the patient.

_____ 2. Health care professionals should not become involved in health care politics.

_____ 3. Controlled substances are drugs that cannot be legally prescribed by physicians or other health care providers.

_____ 4. Frequently returning late from lunch and breaks is a form of dishonesty.

_____ 5. It is acceptable practice to have patient sign-in registers open on the reception desk of a medical office.

_____ 6. Health care professionals must take care when being optimistic with patients about their treatment outcomes.

© 2017 Cengage Learning. All Rights Reserved. May not be scanned, copied or duplicated, or posted to a publicly accessible website, in whole or in part.

_____ 7. Advances in technology have made it difficult to define the meaning of "life."

_____ 8. Withdrawing certain types of artificial life support has become widely acceptable.

_____ 9. Euthanasia means giving comfort measures, such as medication and loving care, as a patient is dying.

_____ 10. Only five states have legalized what is known as mercy killing.

_____ 11. Most dying patients find their approaching death to be depressing and prefer not to talk about it.

_____ 12. Organs can only be taken from individuals who gave permission before their death for their removal.

_____ 13. When many patients are waiting for a limited supply of suitable organs, younger patients are generally given priority for receiving a transplant.

_____ 14. If a child appears to have been physically abused, patient confidentiality prevents health care professionals from reporting suspected abuse.

_____ 15. Patients who are mentally competent have the right to refuse medical treatment.

Multiple Choice

Circle the best answer for each of the following questions. There is only one correct answer to each question.

1. Amy is careful never to reveal information about her patients to anyone who is not entitled to know about their condition. Amy is being __________.

   A. autonomous
   B. discreet
   C. just

2. Violating a patient's right to privacy might result in a __________.

   A. breach of contract
   B. charge of fraud
   C. lawsuit

3. In which of the following situations would giving out information not authorized by a patient be legal?

   A. the patient's injuries were caused by violence, such as a shooting
   B. the patient's sister wants to know details about his condition before traveling to see him
   C. the patient is being cared for at a hospital supported by public funds

4. The guidelines created by the Health Insurance Portability and Accountability Act (HIPAA) are designed to __________

   A. protect the privacy of patient medical records
   B. control rising health care expenses
   C. provide funding for expanded health insurance for the poor

5. While mowing the lawn, Al experiences chest pains and goes to the emergency department of the hospital nearest his home, where he is seen immediately. His actions and those of the treating physician are an example of a/an __________.

   A. breach of contract
   B. express contract
   C. implied contract

© 2017 Cengage Learning. All Rights Reserved. May not be scanned, copied or duplicated, or posted to a publicly accessible website, in whole or in part.

6. Which of the following is NOT a component of a legal contract?

   A. acceptance
   B. offer
   C. consent

7. A medical assistant may be the legal agent of the physician for whom he works. This means that the medical assistant ____________.

   A. has the authority to represent the physician
   B. is required to follow the instructions of the physician
   C. is paid by the physician

8. If a pharmacist makes an error when filling a prescription because he isn't paying full attention to his work, this is an example of ____________.

   A. damages
   B. negligence
   C. respondeat superior

9. A key factor in preventing malpractice lawsuits is to ____________.

   A. develop good interpersonal relationships with patients
   B. ensure that all treatments have successful results
   C. always enter into written contracts with patients

10. Alisa observes a coworker engaging in illegal behavior on the job. She should first ____________.

   A. mind her own business
   B. confront the coworker about her behavior
   C. report what she observes to her supervisor

Short Answer

Read each question. Think about the information presented in the text, and then answer each question.

1. What are five signs that a child may have been physically abused?

   ____

   ____

   ____

2. What are five common considerations used by health care providers to help make decisions about who should receive organ transplants?

   ____

   ____

   ____

3. What are five factors that must be explained to patients when seeking their informed consent for a surgical procedure?

   ____

   ____

   ____

© 2017 Cengage Learning. All Rights Reserved. May not be scanned, copied or duplicated, or posted to a publicly accessible website, in whole or in part.

4. What information is contained in a living will?

____

____

____

5. Some restrictions that insurance providers use to control costs present ethical dilemmas for health care professionals. List three such restrictions.

____

____

____

6. List six forms of elder abuse.

____

____

____

7. What is the purpose of the Occupational Safety and Health Act of 1970?

____

____

____

8. Give four examples of commonly encountered health care fraud.

____

____

____

Completion

Use the words in the list to complete the following statements:

laws	Hippocrates	welfare	responsible
code of ethics	ethical dilemma	consequences	values
ethical principles	technology		

1. The life of a young pregnant woman is in danger due to her pregnancy. Deciding whether to save the mother or the unborn child is an example of a/an _______________.
2. The _______________ of a society are influenced by its history and the religions practiced by its members.
3. The oath developed over 2000 years ago to guide the conduct of physicians was developed by _______________.
4. Advances in medical _______________ have presented today's health care community with many new ethical problems.
5. Most organizations for health care professionals have developed a/an _______________ to guide the conduct of their members.
6. The belief an individual holds about the importance of friendship is influenced by his _______________.

© 2017 Cengage Learning. All Rights Reserved. May not be scanned, copied or duplicated, or posted to a publicly accessible website, in whole or in part.

7. Societies create ______________ based on their ethical principles in order to enforce the behavior that supports these principles.
8. The American legal system is based on the belief that individuals should be __________ for their own actions.
9. Well-intentioned laws sometimes have unintended ______________ that create rather than solve problems.
10. There is sometimes a conflict between the ______________ of patients and the laws and rules that health care professionals must follow.

Critical Thinking

Read each scenario. Think about the information presented in the text, and then answer each question.

1. Carolyn is a physical therapy assistant who has been visiting the home of Mr. Sterns, an 82-year-old man, twice a week. She has noticed that his appearance has deteriorated recently and that he seems unclean with an unwashed odor. He also seems nervous with Carolyn when his son Harold is present.

   A. What might be the problem with Mr. Sterns?

   ____

   ____

   ____

   B. If his situation gets worse and he tells Carolyn he is afraid of his son, what should she do?

   ____

   ____

   ____

2. Craig Samuels has become a frequent repeat visitor to the clinic in which Erin is a medical assistant. Craig complains of various pains and always asks for a prescription for pain medication.

   A. What might be Craig's real reason for visiting the clinic?

   ____

   ____

   ____

   B. What should Erin do?

   ____

   ____

   ____

   C. How does the government control medications such as those that are prescribed for pain?

   ____

   ____

   ____

© 2017 Cengage Learning. All Rights Reserved. May not be scanned, copied or duplicated, or posted to a publicly accessible website, in whole or in part.

UNIT 2
The Language of Health Care

© 2017 Cengage Learning. All Rights Reserved. May not be scanned, copied or duplicated, or posted to a publicly accessible website, in whole or in part.

CHAPTER 4

Medical Terminology

LEARNING OBJECTIVES

Studying and applying the material in this chapter will help you to:

- Understand the importance of being able to write, read, and communicate using medical terminology.
- Identify common roots and combining forms, suffixes, and prefixes.
- Break down medical terms into their component parts and interpret the terms correctly.
- Use the spelling and pronunciation guidelines for medical terms derived from Greek and Latin.
- Define common abbreviations and interpret common symbols.
- Evaluate the features of a medical dictionary to determine its value as a reference for your specialty area.
- Approach the learning of medical terminology by using a variety of study techniques.

© 2017 Cengage Learning. All Rights Reserved. May not be scanned, copied or duplicated, or posted to a publicly accessible website, in whole or in part.

VOCABULARY REVIEW

Definitions

Write the definition of each of the following words or terms.

1. combining form

2. combining vowel

3. consonant

4. medical terminology

5. prefix

6. suffix

7. word part

8. word root

© 2017 Cengage Learning. All Rights Reserved. May not be scanned, copied or duplicated, or posted to a publicly accessible website, in whole or in part.

Matching

Match the following combining forms with their their correct meanings.

_____	1. cephal/o	A.	head
_____	2. cost/o	B.	rib
_____	3. cyt/o	C.	cell
_____	4. cyst/o	D.	gallbladder
_____	5. myel/o	E.	blood
_____	6. pharyng/o	F.	muscle
_____	7. oste/o	G.	spinal cord
_____	8. my/o	H.	urinary bladder
_____	9. hem/o	I.	bone
_____	10. cholecyst/o	J.	throat

CHAPTER REVIEW

Identification

Place an "X" in front of each letter that may be used as a combining vowel.

_____ 1. a

_____ 2. c

_____ 3. g

_____ 4. i

_____ 5. e

_____ 6. o

_____ 7. y

_____ 8. u

_____ 9. x

_____ 10. m

True/False

Indicate whether the following statements are true (T) or false (F).

_____ 1. Hepat/o is a suffix.

_____ 2. Phleb/o means vein.

_____ 3. Cardiomegaly means a smaller than normal sized heart.

_____ 4. Medical terminology should be used when communicating with patients to ensure accurate communications.

_____ 5. Suffixes are word parts that are attached to the end of word roots and combining forms to add to or change their meaning.

© 2017 Cengage Learning. All Rights Reserved. May not be scanned, copied or duplicated, or posted to a publicly accessible website, in whole or in part.

_____ 6. Prefixes are word parts that are attached to the beginning of word roots and combining forms to add to or change their meaning.

_____ 7. When deciphering medical terms it is best to work from the word root, then prefix, and lastly the suffix.

_____ 8. Adip/o, lip/o, and steat/o are all combining forms that mean fat.

_____ 9. Bucco/o is a combining form that means intestine.

_____ 10. Lumpectomy means an incision into a lump.

Multiple Choice

Circle the best answer for each of the following questions. There is only one correct answer to each question.

1. Which of the following combining forms means armpit?
   A. arthr/o
   B. adip/o
   C. axill/o
2. Which of the following parts of a medical term gives the word its main meaning?
   A. root
   B. suffix
   C. prefix
3. Which of the following word roots means stomach?
   A. enter
   B. cardi
   C. gastr
4. Which of the following suffixes means pain?
   A. cide
   B. centesis
   C. algia
5. Which of the following words means a record of the electrical activity of the heart?
   A. electrocardiograph
   B. electrocardiogram
   C. electrocardiography
6. Which of the following descriptions best describes hemiplegia?
   A. numbness of the entire body
   B. burning sensation of the body
   C. paralysis of one side (half) of the body
7. Which of the following prefixes means against?
   A. anti
   B. auto
   C. dys

© 2017 Cengage Learning. All Rights Reserved. May not be scanned, copied or duplicated, or posted to a publicly accessible website, in whole or in part.

8. Which of the following prefixes means after or behind?
   A. post
   B. pre
   C. sub
9. Which of the following abbreviations means twice a day?
   A. a.c.
   B. b.i.d
   C. t.i.d
10. If a patient has an order for NPO and his or her breakfast tray arrives, what is the most appropriate action?
   A. Take the breakfast tray to the patient's room.
   B. Do not take the breakfast tray to the patient's room.
   C. Remove the items that are not liquid and then take it to the patient's room.

Short Answer

Read each question. Think about the information presented in the text, and then answer each question.

1. When pronouncing the words *cell, circulatory,* and *cyst* the *c* sounds like *s*. What medical spelling and pronunciation guideline does this refer to?
____
____
____
2. When pronouncing the word *chronic*. What medical spelling and pronunciation guideline does this refer to?
____
____
____
3. Explain the difference between *gastr* and *gastr/o.*
____
____
____
4. Describe the difference between appendicitis and appendectomy.
____
____
____
5. How is the plural usually formed when the term ends in *is*?
____
____
____

© 2017 Cengage Learning. All Rights Reserved. May not be scanned, copied or duplicated, or posted to a publicly accessible website, in whole or in part.

6. What is the recommended procedure to follow when deciphering medical terms?

____

____

____

7. Using medical abbreviations, write that a patient should have his or her vital signs taken four times a day and can be up walking freely, at will and without assistance.

____

____

____

8. If a patient is to be given a medication *p.c.,* when would you administer the medication?

____

____

____

9. Explain the difference between *ASAP* and *stat.* Which is the most urgent?

____

____

____

10. The plural for *ganglion* is *ganglia.* Write the guideline to making plural forms that this follows.

____

____

____

Completion

Use the words in the list to complete the following statements.

arteri/o	ren/o or nephr/o	viv/o
lapar/o	otomy	cide
emia	derm/o or dermat/o	
ven/o or phleb/o	larygn/o	

1. A combining form that means vein is ___________.
2. A combining form that means artery is ___________.
3. A combining form that means life is ___________.
4. A combining form that means abdominal wall is ___________.
5. A combining form that means voice box or larynx is ___________.
6. A combining form that means kidneys is ___________.
7. A combining form that means skin is ___________.

© 2017 Cengage Learning. All Rights Reserved. May not be scanned, copied or duplicated, or posted to a publicly accessible website, in whole or in part.

8. A suffix that means to kill or destroy is ___________.
9. A suffix that means surgical incision is ___________.
10. A suffix that means blood is ___________.

Critical Thinking Scenarios

Read each scenario. Think about the information presented in the text, and then answer each question.

1. Janet, age 45, has been feeling unusually tired and has noted an unexplained weight gain. She goes to her provider, who determines she has hypothyroidism.

   A. What does hypothyroidism mean?

   ____

   ____

   ____

   B. What does hyperthyroidism mean?

   ____

   ____

   ____

2. Bob, age 56, was seen by his provider for intestinal problems. When he arrived home, he decided to research a word his provider used which sounded like "ILL ee um."

   A. There are two medical terms that are pronounced "ILL ee um." What are they?

   ____

   ____

   ____

   B. What does each term mean?

   ____

   ____

   ____

   C. Which term was the most likely one the provider was using?

   ____

   ____

   ____

© 2017 Cengage Learning. All Rights Reserved. May not be scanned, copied or duplicated, or posted to a publicly accessible website, in whole or in part.

CHAPTER 5

Medical Math

LEARNING OBJECTIVES

Studying and applying the material in this chapter will help you to:

- Understand how math anxiety prevents comfort and competence with calculations.
- Perform basic math calculations on whole numbers, decimals, fractions, percentages, and ratios.
- Convert between the following numerical forms: decimals, fractions, percentages, and ratios.
- Round off numbers correctly.
- Solve mathematical equivalency problems with proportions.
- Express time using the 24-hour clock (military time).
- Express numbers using Roman numerals.
- Estimate angles from a reference plane.
- Use household, metric, and apothecary units to express length, volume, and weight.
- Know equivalencies for converting among the household, metric, and apothecary systems of measurement.
- Convert between the Fahrenheit and Celsius temperature scales.

© 2017 Cengage Learning. All Rights Reserved. May not be scanned, copied or duplicated, or posted to a publicly accessible website, in whole or in part.

VOCABULARY REVIEW

Matching

Match the following terms with their correct definitions.

_____	1. metric system	A.	a method of telling time that is based on a 24-hour clock
_____	2. military time	B.	a method used to express a whole or part of a whole; the whole is written as 100%
_____	3. nomenclature	C.	a method used to express the strength of a solution; it represents how many parts of one element are added in relationship to the parts of another element
_____	4. percentages	D.	a numbering system based on I (1), V (5), X (10), L (50), C (100), D (500), and M (1000)
_____	5. proportion	E.	a mathematical statement of equality between two ratios
_____	6. ratio	F.	method of naming
_____	7. reciprocal	G.	a real or imaginary flat surface from which an angle is measured
_____	8. reference plane	H.	rules that determine whether a number is changed to zero, increased, or remains the same when digits are dropped from the right side
_____	9. Roman numerals	I.	the traditional numbers we use to count (1, 2, 3…)
_____	10. rounding numbers	J.	a measurement system based on 10s; basic units are length (meter), volume (liter), and weight (gram)
_____	11. whole numbers	K.	a fraction that has been "turned upside down" during the process of dividing fractions

Word Fill

Complete the following sentences by filling in the missing words.

angles	apothecary system	centigrade (C) scale	decimal system
degrees	estimating	Fahrenheit (F) scale	fraction
household system	improper fraction	math anxiety	

1. The __________ is a measurement system that is used infrequently except for a measurement of weight (grain).
2. __________ are units of measurement used in angles, temperature readings, and depth of burns.
3. The __________ is a linear arrangement of numbers based on units of 10, containing a point to separate the whole number from the fractional part of a number (e.g., 2.5).

© 2017 Cengage Learning. All Rights Reserved. May not be scanned, copied or duplicated, or posted to a publicly accessible website, in whole or in part.

4. The ___________ is a method used to express numbers that are not whole numbers; it has a numerator and a denominator.
5. The ___________ is a measurement system based on common household items used to measure length, volume, and weight.
6. ___________ are the amount of variance from a reference plane expressed in degrees.
7. ___________ is a measurement of temperature based on a freezing point of 32° and a boiling point of 212°.
8. A/An ___________ is a fraction that has a numerator that is larger than the denominator.
9. ___________ is expressing the approximate answer.
10. ___________ is a strong negative reaction to math that interferes with the ability to concentrate, learn, and perform math calculations.
11. ___________ is a measurement of temperature based on a freezing point of 0° and a boiling point of 100°.

CHAPTER REVIEW

Identification

Place an "X" in front of the following activities that might require math calculations.

_____ 1. administering medications

_____ 2. recording height and weight

_____ 3. tracking intake and output

_____ 4. billing tasks

_____ 5. performing lab tests

_____ 6. mixing solutions

_____ 7. assisting in surgery

_____ 8. providing therapeutic services

_____ 9. taking vital signs

_____ 10. documenting in a patient's chart

True/False

Indicate whether the following statements are true (T) or false (F).

_____ 1. Work in health care requires the use of math skills to measure and perform various types of calculations.

_____ 2. Dividing fractions requires the dividing fraction to be inverted (turned upside down). The new, upside-down fraction is called an improper fraction.

_____ 3. Rounding 135 to the nearest whole number would be 135.

_____ 4. Rounding 274.56 to the nearest whole number would be 275.

_____ 5. The military time of 1230 would be expressed as 12:30 a.m. in traditional time.

© 2017 Cengage Learning. All Rights Reserved. May not be scanned, copied or duplicated, or posted to a publicly accessible website, in whole or in part.

_____ 6. The Roman numeral XXVIII is 27 in Arabic numbers.

_____ 7. A needle held perpendicular to the reference plane would be at a 180 degree angle.

_____ 8. In the household measurement system, there are three teaspoons in one tablespoon.

_____ 9. To convert grams to kilograms, you would add three zeros.

_____ 10. To convert grams to centigrams, you would add three zeros.

Multiple Choice

Circle the best answer for each of the following questions. There is only one correct answer to each question.

1. Which of the following is true about math anxiety?
   A. it is a learned behavior
   B. it is an inherited trait
   C. it cannot be overcome
2. How is 1.60 read?
   A. one and sixty-tenths
   B. one and six-tenths
   C. one and sixty-hundredths
3. Which is the proper way to write three milligrams?
   A. 3.0 mg
   B. 0.3 mg
   C. 3 mg
4. Which of the following abbreviations is acceptable to use in medical documentation?
   A. U
   B. mL
   C. cc
5. What is the result of multiplying 1.5 times 1.125?
   A. 0.16875
   B. 168.75
   C. 1.6875
6. What is the result of adding 1/2 to 1/3?
   A. 2/5
   B. 5/6
   C. 1/6
7. What would the decimal 0.75 be converted to when expressed as a fraction?
   A. 3/4
   B. 75%
   C. 7.5
8. What is the military time for 4 p.m.?
   A. 0400
   B. 0160
   C. 1600

© 2017 Cengage Learning. All Rights Reserved. May not be scanned, copied or duplicated, or posted to a publicly accessible website, in whole or in part.

9. How many ounces are in one cup?
   A. 4
   B. 8
   C. 16
10. A child measures 19 inches in length. How many centimeters is this?
   A. 47.5
   B. 7.6
   C. 38

Short Answer

Read each question. Think about the information presented in the text, and then answer each question.

1. Why is it critical that health care workers strive for 100% accuracy in math?

____

____

____

2. What is math anxiety? Can it be overcome?

____

____

____

3. What is the number 345.345 rounded to the nearest tens and the nearest tenths?

____

____

____

4. If a patient is 66 inches tall, how would that be expressed in feet?

____

____

____

5. What is the value of estimating in calculations?

____

____

____

6. What are the seven key numerals used with Roman numerals and what value does each represent?

____

____

____

© 2017 Cengage Learning. All Rights Reserved. May not be scanned, copied or duplicated, or posted to a publicly accessible website, in whole or in part.

7. What is the nomenclature in the metric system for distance/length, capacity/volume, and mass/weight?

8. What do the prefixes *kilo, centi,* and *milli* mean?

9. What are the primary approximate equivalents between measuring systems?

10. How do the boiling and freezing points between the Fahrenheit (F) and Celsius (C) systems compare?

Critical Thinking Scenarios

Read each scenario. Think about the information presented in the text, and then answer each question.

1. Mr. John Brown says he has medication that states he is to take 15 milliliters every day. He is confused by the instructions and asks you to clarify.

   A. How many milliliters are in 1 teaspoon?

   B. How many milliliters are in 1 tablespoon?

   C. What amount would you recommend for him to take?

© 2017 Cengage Learning. All Rights Reserved. May not be scanned, copied or duplicated, or posted to a publicly accessible website, in whole or in part.

2. A patient states that she weighs 125 pounds and wants to know how that converts to kilograms.

   A. What is the equivalent between the two systems?

   B. What are the abbreviations for pounds and kilograms?

   C. How much does the patient weigh in kilograms rounded to the nearest tenth?

© 2017 Cengage Learning. All Rights Reserved. May not be scanned, copied or duplicated, or posted to a publicly accessible website, in whole or in part.

UNIT 3
The Human Body

© 2017 Cengage Learning. All Rights Reserved. May not be scanned, copied or duplicated, or posted to a publicly accessible website, in whole or in part.

CHAPTER 6

Organization of the Human Body

LEARNING OBJECTIVES

Studying and applying the material in this chapter will help you to:

- Explain the meaning of homeostasis.
- Name the levels in the structural organization of the body.
- Name and explain the functions of the main cellular components.
- Name and describe the four primary types of tissues.
- Describe the anatomical position.
- Identify and describe the location of the three directional body planes.
- Use directional terms to describe various locations on the body.
- Name the main body cavities and what structures are found in each.
- Identify the abdominal regions and quadrants.

© 2017 Cengage Learning. All Rights Reserved. May not be scanned, copied or duplicated, or posted to a publicly accessible website, in whole or in part.

VOCABULARY REVIEW

Matching 1

Match the following terms with their correct definitions.

_____	1. lateral	A.	away from the center of the body (toward the sides)
_____	2. medial	B.	anatomical term meaning away from the center
_____	3. midsagittal plane	C.	located in the chest; contains the heart, lungs, and major blood vessels
_____	4. organ	D.	passes through the midline and divides the body vertically into equal right and left portions
_____	5. pelvic cavity	E.	groups of cells with a similar function
_____	6. peripheral	F.	consists of the cranial and spinal cavity; protects the structures of the nervous system; also called dorsal body cavity
_____	7. posterior (dorsal)	G.	near or close to the body surface
_____	8. posterior body cavity	H.	toward the midline or center of body
_____	9. proximal	I.	divides the body horizontally into top and bottom portions
_____	10. spinal cavity	J.	located within the spinal column; contains the spinal cord
_____	11. superficial	K.	above
_____	12. superior	L.	located in the lower abdomen; contains the urinary bladder, rectum, and reproductive organs
_____	13. tissue	M.	closer to the reference point
_____	14. thoracic cavity	N.	toward the back of the body
_____	15. transverse plane	O.	the combination of two or more types of tissues that work together to perform a specific body function

Word Fill

Complete the following sentences by filling in the missing words.

abdominal cavity	anatomical position	anterior (ventral)	anterior body cavity
apex	base	body system	caudal
cell	cephalic (cranial)	cranial cavity	deep
distal	frontal plane	homeostasis	inferior

1. ______________________ is at the top (highest point).
2. ______________________ is closer to the coccyx (lower back).

© 2017 Cengage Learning. All Rights Reserved. May not be scanned, copied or duplicated, or posted to a publicly accessible website, in whole or in part.

3. ______________________ is the tendency of a cell or the whole organism to maintain a state of balance.
4. ______________________ is when the body as viewed in a full upright position (standing), with the arms relaxed at the sides of the body, palms facing forward, feet pointed forward, and the eyes directed straight ahead.
5. A ______________________ is a combination of two or more organs to provide a major body function.
6. ______________________ is farther from the reference base point.
7. The ______________________ divides the body vertically into front and back portions.
8. ______________________ is at the bottom (lowest point).
9. The ______________________ contains the stomach, intestines, liver, gallbladder, pancreas, and spleen.
10. ______________________ means farther from the body surface.
11. The ______________________ is located in the skull; it contains the brain.
12. The ______________________ consists of the thoracic, abdominal, and pelvic cavities; protects the internal organs; and is also called the ventral body cavity.
13. A ______________________ is the smallest living structure of the body.
14. ______________________ is closer to the head.
15. ______________________ is below.
16. ______________________ is toward the front of body.

CHAPTER REVIEW

Identification

Place an "X" in front of the cell components that are organelles.

_____ 1. endoplasmic reticulum

_____ 2. centrioles

_____ 3. cell membrane

_____ 4. nucleus

_____ 5. cytoplasm

_____ 6. vesicle

_____ 7. protoplasm

_____ 8. Golgi apparatus

_____ 9. ribosomes

_____ 10. lysosome

_____ 11. mitochondrion

© 2017 Cengage Learning. All Rights Reserved. May not be scanned, copied or duplicated, or posted to a publicly accessible website, in whole or in part.

True/False

Indicate whether the following statements are true (T) or false (F).

_____ 1. Adjustments made to maintain homeostasis occur without our conscious awareness.

_____ 2. The posterior (dorsal) cavity includes the thoracic, abdominal, and pelvic cavities.

_____ 3. The nucleus controls the activity of the cell.

_____ 4. The umbilicus is on the anterior surface of the body.

_____ 5. When standing in the anatomical position, the elbows are on the posterior (dorsal) side of the body.

_____ 6. The elbow is proximal to the shoulder.

_____ 7. The breasts are caudal to the waist.

_____ 8. In the anatomical position, the thumb is medial to the other fingers.

_____ 9. An abrasion below the armpit would be on the lateral side of the body.

_____ 10. The epigastric region is located superior to the hypogastric region.

Matching 2

Match the following types of cells with their correct functions. Each function is used only once.

_____	1. bone cells	A. communication
_____	2. nerve cells	B. protection
_____	3. skin cells	C. oxygen transportation
_____	4. muscle cells	D. movement
_____	5. red blood cells	E. support

Ordering

Place the following structures in the order of the smallest to the largest level. Put a numeral 1 before the smallest structure, a 2 before the next, and so on.

_____ organs

_____ tissues

_____ human body as a whole

_____ cell

_____ body (organ) systems

© 2017 Cengage Learning. All Rights Reserved. May not be scanned, copied or duplicated, or posted to a publicly accessible website, in whole or in part.

Labeling

Assign the major components of the cell from the list below to the appropriate places on the figure.

Figure 6–1

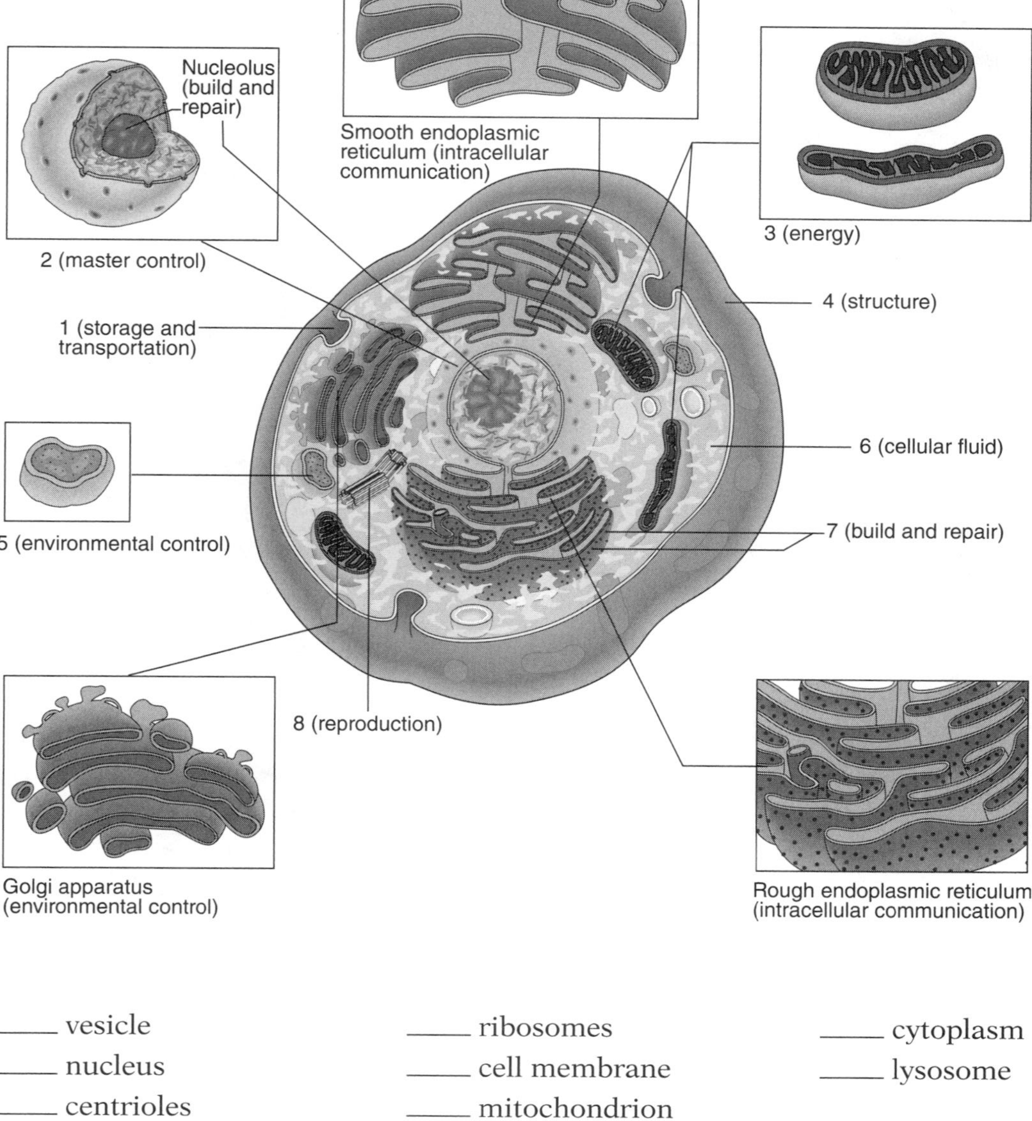

_____ vesicle	_____ ribosomes	_____ cytoplasm
_____ nucleus	_____ cell membrane	_____ lysosome
_____ centrioles	_____ mitochondrion	

© 2017 Cengage Learning. All Rights Reserved. May not be scanned, copied or duplicated, or posted to a publicly accessible website, in whole or in part.

Assign the directional terms from the following list to the appropriate places on the figures.

Figure 6–2a and 6–2b

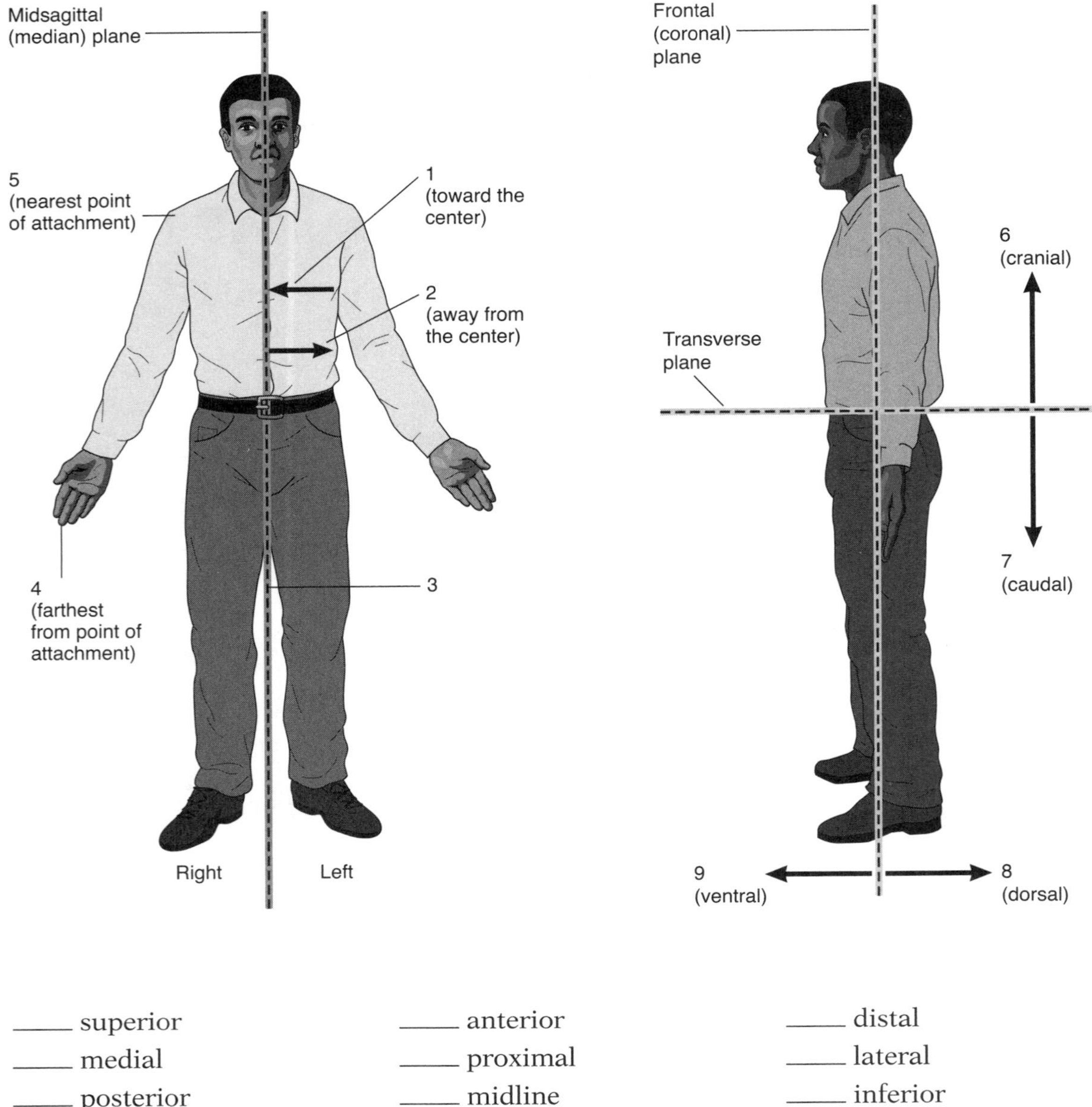

_____ superior
_____ medial
_____ posterior
_____ anterior
_____ proximal
_____ midline
_____ distal
_____ lateral
_____ inferior

© 2017 Cengage Learning. All Rights Reserved. May not be scanned, copied or duplicated, or posted to a publicly accessible website, in whole or in part.

Assign the body cavities from the following list to the appropriate places on the figure.

Figure 6–3

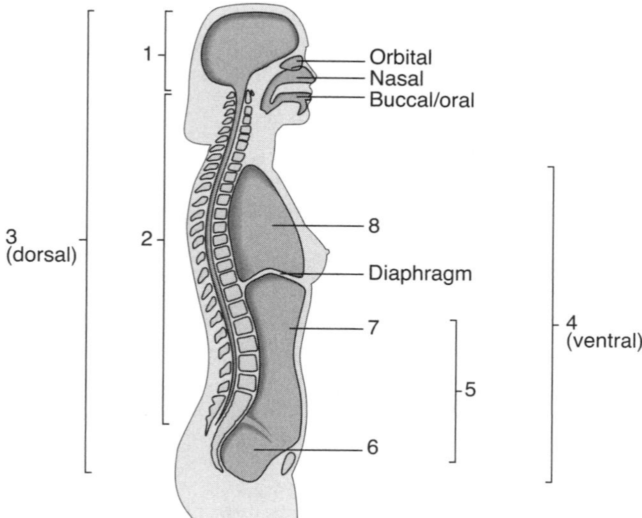

____ posterior
____ abdominopelvic
____ thoracic
____ anterior
____ spinal
____ cranial
____ abdominal
____ pelvic

Assign the regions and quadrants listed below to the appropriate places on the figures.

Figure 6–4a and 6–4b

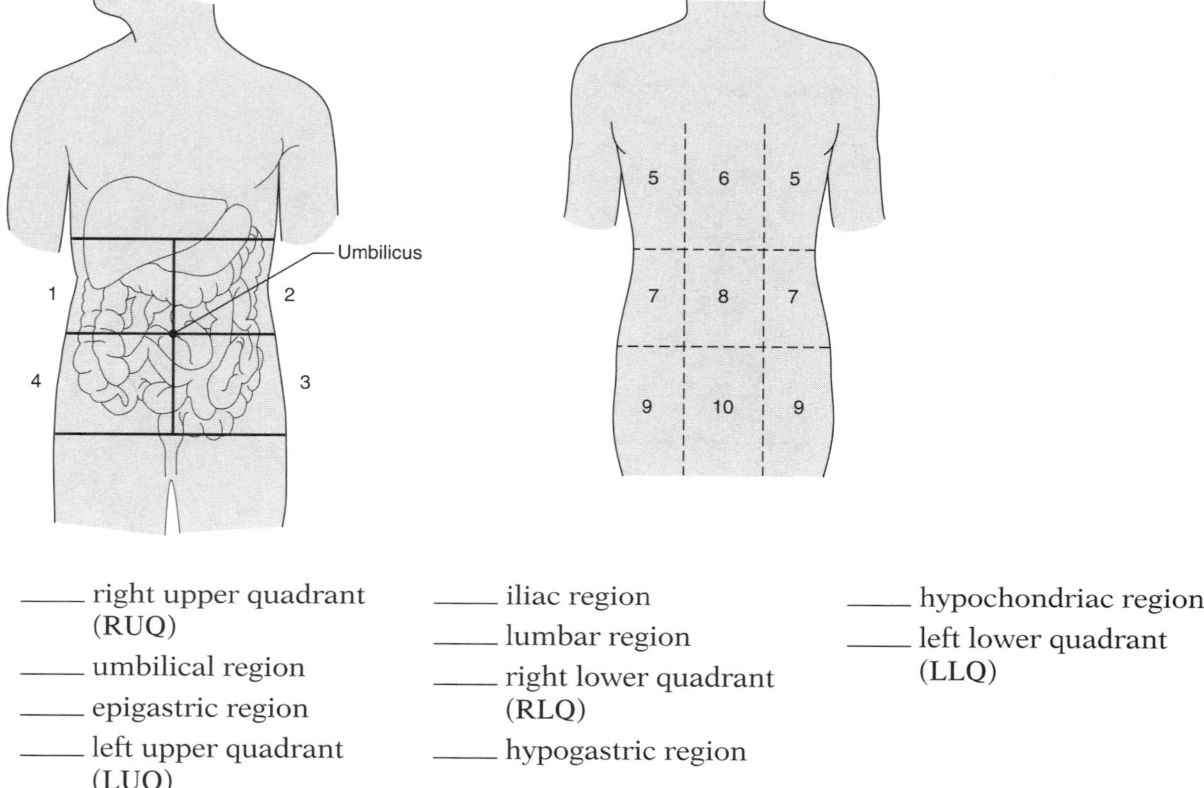

____ right upper quadrant (RUQ)
____ umbilical region
____ epigastric region
____ left upper quadrant (LUQ)
____ iliac region
____ lumbar region
____ right lower quadrant (RLQ)
____ hypogastric region
____ hypochondriac region
____ left lower quadrant (LLQ)

© 2017 Cengage Learning. All Rights Reserved. May not be scanned, copied or duplicated, or posted to a publicly accessible website, in whole or in part.

Critical Thinking Scenarios

Read each scenario. Think about the information presented in the text, and then answer each question.

1. Mr. Travis Weathers arrives in the emergency department with complaints of severe abdominal pain after an accident. When asks where the pain is he rubs his hand clear across the abdomen above the umbilicus.

   A. Using the four quadrant model, how would you describe this location?

   ____

   ____

   ____

   B. Is the pain on the anterior (ventral) or posterior (dorsal) side of the body?

   ____

   ____

   ____

   C. Would lateral or medial be used in this description?

   ____

   ____

   ____

2. Ms. Matilda Bush is taken to surgery after sustaining multiple abrasions from a motorcycle accident. It is necessary to anesthetize her in order to remove the gravel that has been ground into her skin. She also has a bruised area that extends from the shoulder to the elbow of the left arm. You also note there is moderate edema of her feet and ankles.

   A. Would her injuries be considered superficial or deep?

   ____

   ____

   ____

   B. How would you describe the location of the bruise?

   ____

   ____

   ____

   C. How would you describe the edema?

   ____

   ____

   ____

© 2017 Cengage Learning. All Rights Reserved. May not be scanned, copied or duplicated, or posted to a publicly accessible website, in whole or in part.

CHAPTER 7

Structure and Function of the Human Body

LEARNING OBJECTIVES

Studying and applying the material in this chapter will help you to:

- Understand and explain the difference between anatomy, physiology, and pathophysiology.
- Define what determines a state of wellness as opposed to illness.
- Describe the primary anatomical features and physiological actions of the systems for movement and protection of the body.
- Name and demonstrate the movements made possible by joints.
- Describe the primary anatomical features and physiological actions of the systems for providing energy and for removing waste from the body.
- Describe the primary anatomical features and physiological actions of the systems for sensing and for coordinating and controlling the body.
- Describe the primary anatomical features and physiological actions of the systems for producing new life.
- Name common diseases or disorders associated with each system.
- Describe the behaviors and actions for each body system that promote health and prevent major diseases and disorders.

© 2017 Cengage Learning. All Rights Reserved. May not be scanned, copied or duplicated, or posted to a publicly accessible website, in whole or in part.

VOCABULARY REVIEW

Definitions

Write the definition of each of the following words or terms.

1. anatomy

2. diagnosis

3. diagnostic procedures

4. diseases

5. etiology

6. illness

7. objective

8. pathophysiology

© 2017 Cengage Learning. All Rights Reserved. May not be scanned, copied or duplicated, or posted to a publicly accessible website, in whole or in part.

Matching 1

Match the following terms with their correct definitions.

_____	1. physiology	A.	when the body is in a state of homeostasis
_____	2. prevention (of disease)	B.	something that is dependent on or takes place in a person's mind, and cannot be directly observed
_____	3. prognosis	C.	prediction of the possible outcome of a disease and the potential for recovery
_____	4. signs and symptoms	D.	medications or procedures used to control or cure a disease or injury
_____	5. subjective	E.	not a precise disease but a group of related signs and symptoms
_____	6. syndrome	F.	the objective evidence observed by the health care worker and the subjective data reported by patients about their condition
_____	7. wellness	G.	the study of the functions (how and why something works) of an organism
_____	8. treatment	H.	behaviors that promote health and prevent disease

CHAPTER REVIEW

Identification

Place an "X" in front of the bones that are part of the axial skeleton.

_____ 1. hyoid

_____ 2. feet

_____ 3. skull

_____ 4. inner ear

_____ 5. pelvis

_____ 6. hands

_____ 7. spinal column

_____ 8. legs

_____ 9. arms

_____ 10. ribs

_____ 11. sternum

© 2017 Cengage Learning. All Rights Reserved. May not be scanned, copied or duplicated, or posted to a publicly accessible website, in whole or in part.

True/False Rewrite

Please rewrite the bold part of the sentence to make the statement true.

1. The **atrioventricular node (AV node)** is known as the natural pacemaker of the heart.

2. The **dermis** is the outer layer of the skin.

3. **Platelets** are the liquid part of the blood, consisting mostly of water.

4. The second essential transportation system of the body is the **endocrine** system.

5. **Leukemia** results when the blood has an inadequate amount of hemoglobin, red blood cells, or both.

6. The **nervous** system provides energy for the body by processing food.

7. **An ulcer** is a condition in which the lining of the abdominal cavity becomes inflamed.

8. **Edema** is a disease.

© 2017 Cengage Learning. All Rights Reserved. May not be scanned, copied or duplicated, or posted to a publicly accessible website, in whole or in part.

9. The **conjunctiva** produce tears for cleaning and moisturizing the eyes.

____

____

____

10. The **cochlea** are three tiny, delicate bones that form a chain to carry and amplify sound vibrations from the eardrum.

____

____

____

Multiple Choice

Circle the best answer for each of the following questions. There is only one correct answer to each question.

1. Which of the following is a lateral curvature of the spine?

   A. kyphosis
   B. lordosis
   C. scoliosis

2. Which of the following is an inward curvature of the lumbar area?

   A. kyphosis
   B. lordosis
   C. scoliosis

3. Which of the following is a rounded bowing of the thoracic area?

   A. kyphosis
   B. lordosis
   C. scoliosis

4. Which of the following is the medical term for the throat?

   A. larynx
   B. pharynx
   C. trachea

5. Which of the following structures have villi?

   A. throat
   B. stomach
   C. small intestine

6. Which of the following is also known as myopia?

   A. nearsightedness
   B. farsightedness
   C. glaucoma

© 2017 Cengage Learning. All Rights Reserved. May not be scanned, copied or duplicated, or posted to a publicly accessible website, in whole or in part.

7. Which of the following is part of the peripheral nervous system?

   A. brain
   B. spinal cord
   C. cranial nerves

8. Which of the following conditions is caused by excessive thyroid hormones?

   A. hyperthyroidism
   B. hypothyroidism
   C. acromegaly

9. Which of the following structures connects the bladder to the exterior of the body?

   A. ureter
   B. urethra
   C. uvula

10. Which of the following is an inflammation of the testes?

    A. phimosis
    B. epididymitis
    C. orchitis

Matching 2

Match the following terms with their correct definitions.

_____	1. phimosis	A.	tumors of the uterus
_____	2. dementia	B.	excessive hormone production of the adrenal cortex
_____	3. encephalitis	C.	tightness of the foreskin over the end of the penis
_____	4. macular degeneration	D.	abnormal electrical impulses in the neurons
_____	5. glaucoma	E.	infection of the middle ear
_____	6. diabetes mellitus	F.	loss of memory and impairment of mental function
_____	7. otitis media	G.	infection of the brain
_____	8. Cushing's syndrome	H.	increased pressure in the eye
_____	9. epilepsy	I.	disorder of the retina
_____	10. fibroid tumors	J.	caused by inadequate insulin

© 2017 Cengage Learning. All Rights Reserved. May not be scanned, copied or duplicated, or posted to a publicly accessible website, in whole or in part.

Completion

Use the words in the list to complete the following statements:

flat	short	periosteum	medullary canal
irregular	red marrow	cartilage	long
diaphysis	epiphyses		

1. The __________ is the center cavity of a long bone containing yellow marrow.
2. The __________ is the portion that runs between the ends of the bone.
3. The __________ are the ends of the bone (proximal and distal).
4. The __________ is the white, fibrous layer that covers the outside of bone; it contains blood, lymph vessels, and nerves.
5. The __________ is the part of the bone that manufactures the red blood cells (RBCs), which carry oxygen, and the white blood cells (WBCs), which protect the body from infections.
6. The __________ is the elastic connective tissue that covers the end of the bones and functions as a cushion between bones.
7. __________ bones are longer than they are wide (e.g., humerus, femur, fingers and toes).
8. __________ bones are similar in length and width (e.g., carpals and tarsals).
9. __________ bones have two layers with space between them (e.g., cranium, ribs, and pelvis).
10. __________ bones are those that do not fit into any other category (e.g., vertebrae and patella).

Ordering 1

Place the following list of electrical structures and cardiac responses in the order in which they would occur. Put a numeral 1 before the structure where the electrical impulse originates, a 2 before the next, and so on.

_____ left and right atria contract

_____ bundle of His

_____ atrioventricular node (AV node)

_____ sinoatrial node (SA node)

_____ right and left bundle fibers

_____ right and left ventricles contract

_____ Purkinje fibers

© 2017 Cengage Learning. All Rights Reserved. May not be scanned, copied or duplicated, or posted to a publicly accessible website, in whole or in part.

Ordering 2

Place the following list in the proper sequence to represent the flow of the blood through the cardiovascular system. Put a numeral 1 before the structures that bring the blood from the body to the heart, 2 before the next, and so on.

_____ 1. right atrium

_____ 2. left ventricle

_____ 3. superior and inferior vena cavae

_____ 4. pulmonary veins

_____ 5. left atrium

_____ 6. pulmonary arteries

_____ 7. right ventricle

_____ 8. lungs

_____ 9. aorta

Labeling

Assign the labels from the list below to the appropriate places on the figure.

Figure 7–1

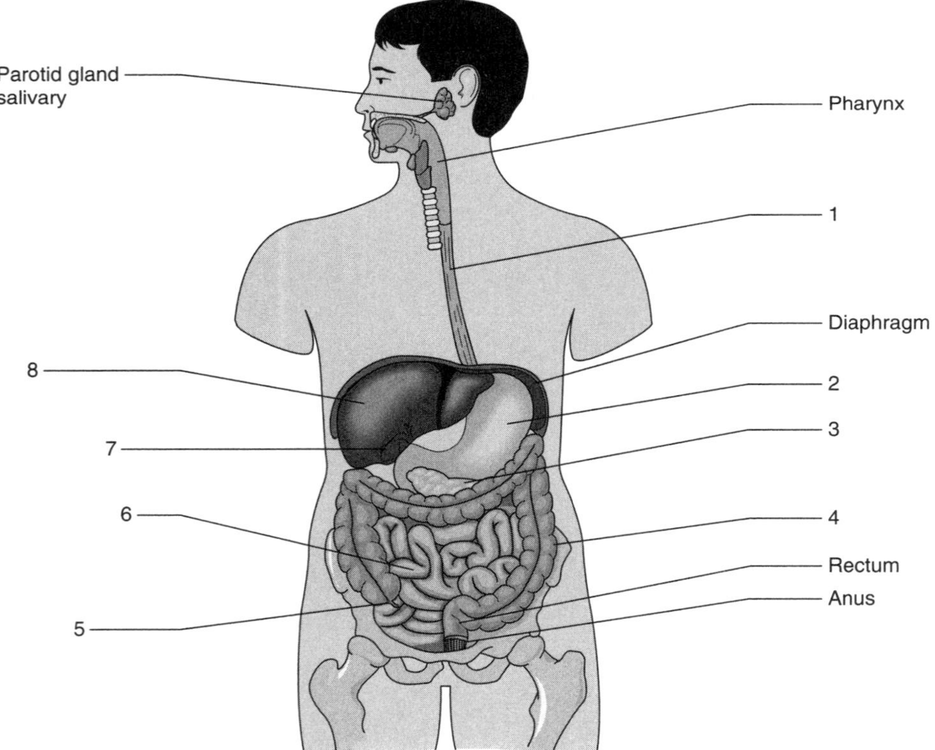

1. _____ gall bladder
2. _____ esophagus
3. _____ pancreas
4. _____ liver
5. _____ large intestine
6. _____ small intestine
7. _____ stomach
8. _____ appendix

© 2017 Cengage Learning. All Rights Reserved. May not be scanned, copied or duplicated, or posted to a publicly accessible website, in whole or in part.

Assign the labels from the list below to the appropriate places on the figure.

Figure 7–2

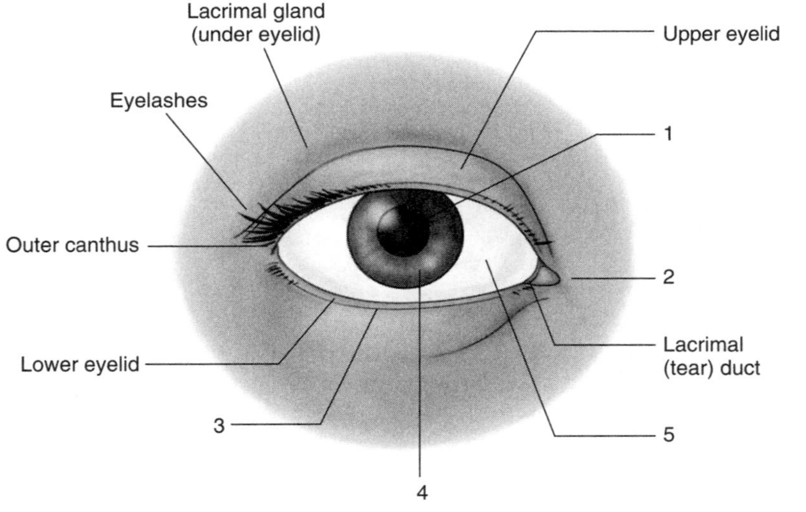

1. _____ sclera
2. _____ pupil
3. _____ conjunctiva
4. _____ iris
5. _____ inner canthus

Assign the labels from the list below to the appropriate places on the figure.

Figure 7–3

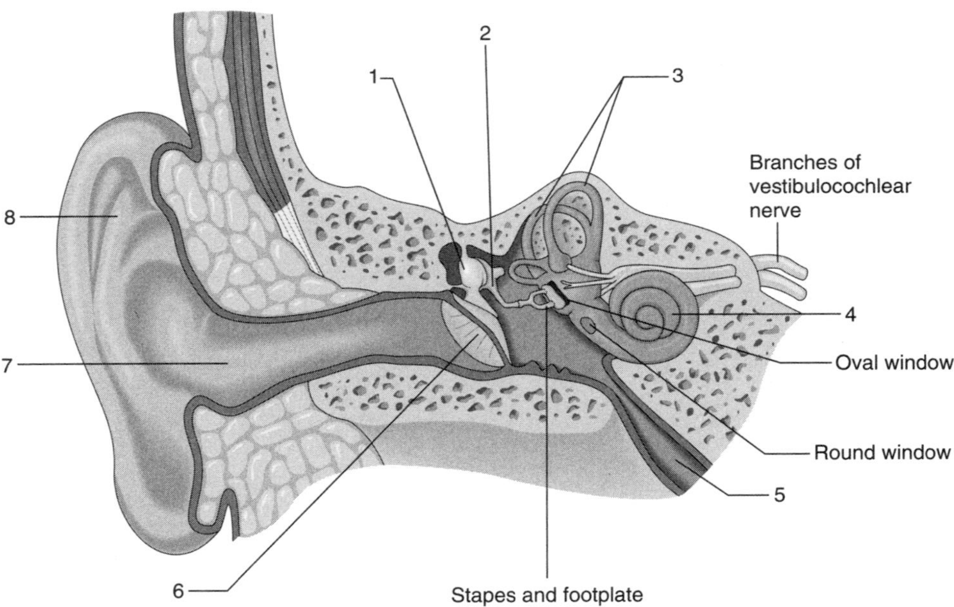

1. _____ external auditory canal
2. _____ incus
3. _____ cochlea
4. _____ auditory (Eustachian) tube
5. _____ tympanic membrane
6. _____ auricle
7. _____ malleus
8. _____ semicircular canals

© 2017 Cengage Learning. All Rights Reserved. May not be scanned, copied or duplicated, or posted to a publicly accessible website, in whole or in part.

Assign the labels from the list below to the appropriate places on the figure.

Figure 7–4

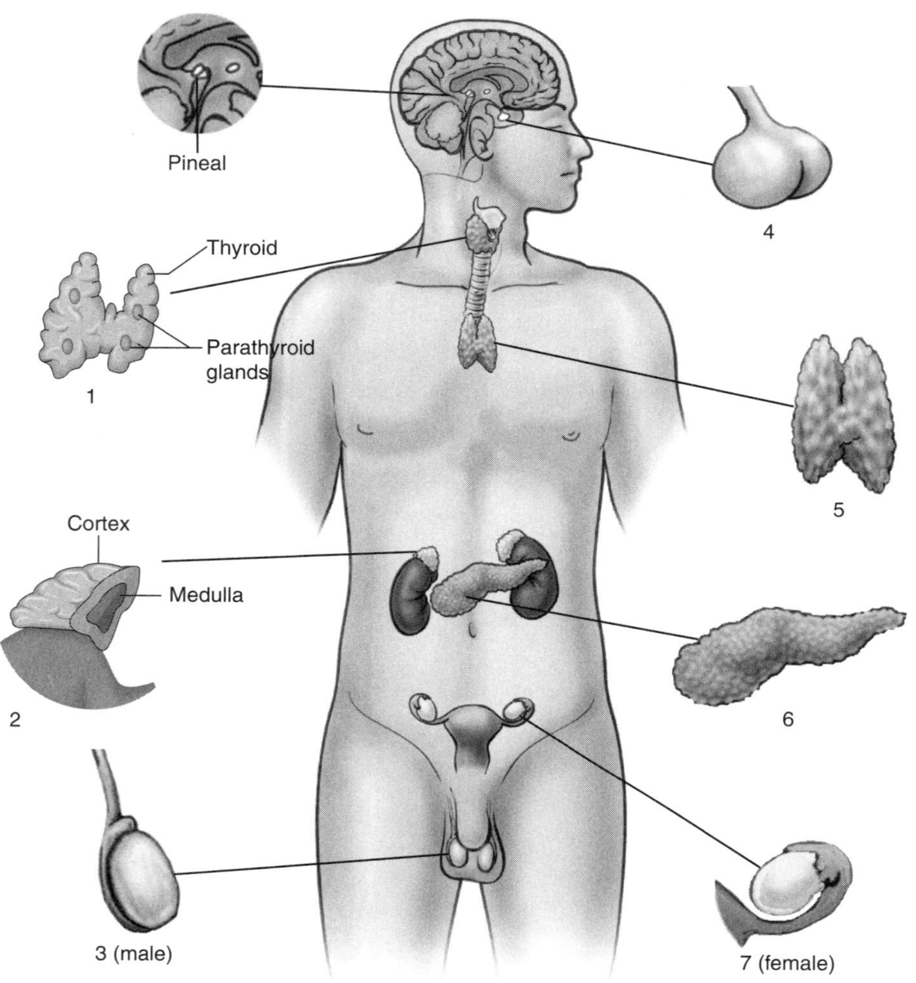

1. _____ pancreas
2. _____ pituitary
3. _____ thymus
4. _____ adrenal
5. _____ testis
6. _____ ovary
7. _____ parathyroid

© 2017 Cengage Learning. All Rights Reserved. May not be scanned, copied or duplicated, or posted to a publicly accessible website, in whole or in part.

Critical Thinking Scenarios

Read each scenario. Think about the information presented in the text, and then answer each question.

1. Juanita Barber thought she was just having a chest cold, but when she started to have increasing difficulty breathing she went to the health care provider. She has a chest X-ray done and is informed there is atelectasis in the left lower lobe and the diagnosis is pneumonia.

   A. What is atelectasis and what is the likely cause?

   ____

   ____

   ____

   B. What causes pneumonia?

   ____

   ____

   ____

   C. How many lobes are there in the two lungs?

   ____

   ____

   ____

2. Lam Pham has not been feeling well for some time. A number of tests were run and it was determined he has Hodgkin's disease.

   A. What is Hodgkin's disease?

   ____

   ____

   ____

   B. What system does this disease involve?

   ____

   ____

   ____

   C. What is the function of this system?

   ____

   ____

   ____

© 2017 Cengage Learning. All Rights Reserved. May not be scanned, copied or duplicated, or posted to a publicly accessible website, in whole or in part.

CHAPTER 8

Growth and Development

LEARNING OBJECTIVES

Studying and applying the material in this chapter will help you to:

- Explain the differences between *physical, cognitive,* and *psychosocial* as they relate to growth and development.
- Identify the nine life stages according to the theory of Erik Erikson and the corresponding age span for each.
- Discuss the physical, cognitive, and psychosocial changes that occur at each life stage according to the theory of Erik Erikson.
- Identify the psychosocial developmental tasks to be accomplished according to the theory of Erik Erikson.
- Implement specific approaches to care at each life stage based on a knowledge of growth and development.
- Discuss the main concepts of the developmental theories of Piaget, Kohlberg, and Gilligan.
- Identify and describe the five stages of the dying process.

VOCABULARY

Definitions

Write the definition of each of the following words or terms.

1. chronic illness

____

____

____

2. cognitive development

____

____

____

© 2017 Cengage Learning. All Rights Reserved. May not be scanned, copied or duplicated, or posted to a publicly accessible website, in whole or in part.

3. development

____

____

____

4. growth

____

____

____

Word Fill

Complete the following sentences by filling in the missing words.

Erikson's stages of psychosocial development	Piaget's cognitive stages	physical development	psychosocial development
Gilligan's stages of the ethic of care	life review	stages of dying	
Kohlberg's moral stages	terminal illness		

1. ____________________ is a developmental theory based on the psychosocial challenges that are presented to individuals as they progress through life stages.
2. ____________________ is a developmental theory that includes the caring effect of human relationships.
3. ____________________ is a developmental theory that is concerned only with children.
4. ____________________ is a developmental theory that has six stages classified into three levels, through which one can only progress one stage at a time.
5. ____________________ is an illness from which the patient is expected to die because there is no known cure.
6. ____________________ is the growth of the body, including motor sensory adaptation.
7. ____________________ is telling the events of one's life as a form of self-evaluation and closure as the end of life approaches.
8. The ____________________ are the stages that dying persons may experience as they face the fact of their own death. The five stages are denial, anger, bargaining, depression, and acceptance.
9. ____________________ refers to the emotions, attitudes, and other aspects of the mind, in addition to the individual's interactions and relationships with other members of society.

© 2017 Cengage Learning. All Rights Reserved. May not be scanned, copied or duplicated, or posted to a publicly accessible website, in whole or in part.

CHAPTER REVIEW

Identification 1

Place an "X" in front of the care considerations appropriate to the infancy life stage according to the theory of Erik Erikson.

_____ 1. involve parents in care

_____ 2. use a firm, direct approach

_____ 3. set limits and maintain safety

_____ 4. praise good behavior

_____ 5. cuddle and hug

Identification 2

Place an "X" in front of the care considerations appropriate to the toddler life stage according to the theory of Erik Erikson.

_____ 1. set limits and maintain safety

_____ 2. distract and use a game approach to improve cooperation

_____ 3. use a firm, direct approach

_____ 4. give only one direction at a time and state it simply

_____ 5. give explanations along with the rationale

Identification 3

Place an "X" in front of the care considerations appropriate to the adolescence life stage according to the theory of Erik Erikson.

_____ 1. encourage questions

_____ 2. provide privacy

_____ 3. explore support systems

_____ 4. encourage active learning, thinking, and use of memory skills

_____ 5. don't talk about them where they can overhear the conversation

Identification 4

Place an "X" in front of the care considerations appropriate to the young adulthood life stage according to the theory of Erik Erikson.

_____ 1. use a firm, direct approach

_____ 2. involve parents in care

_____ 3. involve them in the decision-making process

_____ 4. watch body language for clues regarding feelings

_____ 5. define and enforce behavior limits

© 2017 Cengage Learning. All Rights Reserved. May not be scanned, copied or duplicated, or posted to a publicly accessible website, in whole or in part.

Identification 5

Place an "X" in front of the care considerations appropriate to the later adulthood life stage according to the theory of Erik Erikson.

_____ 1. assist with adjustment to new roles

_____ 2. encourage active learning, thinking, and use of memory skills

_____ 3. provide a lot of physical contact

_____ 4. use a firm, direct approach

_____ 5. give only one direction at a time and state it simply

Multiple Choice

Circle the best answer for each of the following questions. There is only one correct answer to each question.

1. What is the infancy age range as defined by Erik Erikson's stages of psychosocial development?

   A. conception to birth
   B. birth to 1 year
   C. birth to 2 years

2. What is the toddler age range as defined by Erik Erikson's stages of psychosocial development?

   A. 6 months to 2 years
   B. 2 to 3 years
   C. 1 to 3 years

3. What is the preschooler age range as defined by Erik Erikson's stages of psychosocial development?

   A. 3 to 6 years
   B. 2 to 5 years
   C. 4 to 7 years

4. What is the school-age child age range as defined by Erik Erikson's stages of psychosocial development?

   A. 7 to 18 years
   B. 6 to 10 years
   C. 6 to 12 years

5. What is the adolescence age range as defined by Erik Erikson's stages of psychosocial development?

   A. 10 to 18 years
   B. 12 to 20 years
   C. 13 to 16 years

6. What is the young adulthood age range as defined by Erik Erikson's stages of psychosocial development?

   A. 20s and 30s
   B. teens and 20s
   C. 18 to 25 years

© 2017 Cengage Learning. All Rights Reserved. May not be scanned, copied or duplicated, or posted to a publicly accessible website, in whole or in part.

7. What is the middle adulthood age range as defined by Erik Erikson's stages of psychosocial development?

   A. 30s and 40s
   B. 40s and 50s
   C. 40 to 65 years

8. What is the later adulthood age range as defined by Erik Erikson's stages of psychosocial development?

   A. over 55 years
   B. over 65 years
   C. over 75 years

9. Which of the following stages of death and dying is usually the first to be experienced?

   A. anger
   B. depression
   C. denial

10. Which of the following developed the stages of death and dying?

    A. Dr. William Thomas
    B. Erik Erikson
    C. Elisabeth Kübler-Ross

Matching

Match the following life stages to Erikson's stages of psychosocial development.

_____	1. infancy	A. generativity vs. stagnation
_____	2. toddler	B. ego integrity vs. despair
_____	3. preschooler	C. initiative vs. guilt
_____	4. school-age child	D. trust vs. mistrust
_____	5. adolescence	E. identity vs. role confusion
_____	6. young adulthood	F. industry vs. inferiority
_____	7. middle adulthood	G. autonomy vs. shame/doubt
_____	8. later adulthood	H. intimacy vs. isolation

Short Answer

Read each question. Think about the information presented in the text, and then answer each question.

1. Who developed the five stages of dying?

   ____

   ____

   ____

© 2017 Cengage Learning. All Rights Reserved. May not be scanned, copied or duplicated, or posted to a publicly accessible website, in whole or in part.

2. What are the five stages of dying?

3. Why can the five stages of dying apply to any form of loss?

4. Do the five stages of dying proceed in a specific sequence?

5. What is a life review?

6. In the stages of dying, what is the denial stage?

7. In the stages of dying, what is the anger stage?

8. In the stages of dying, what is the bargaining stage?

9. In the stages of dying, what is the depression stage?

10. In the stages of dying, what is the acceptance stage?

© 2017 Cengage Learning. All Rights Reserved. May not be scanned, copied or duplicated, or posted to a publicly accessible website, in whole or in part.

Critical Thinking Scenarios

Read each scenario. Think about the information presented in the text, and then answer each question.

1. Ms. Jennifer Chang brings her 5-year-old child to the clinic for a routine checkup.

   A. According to the theory of Erik Erikson, which life stage would this child's age fall within?

   ____

   ____

   ____

   B. According to Erik Erikson's stages of psychosocial development, what developmental stage does this age group address?

   ____

   ____

   ____

   C. According to the theory of Erik Erikson, what care considerations should be considered when working with this age group?

   ____

   ____

   ____

2. Whitney Comb is a retired financial planner. She is 80 years old and is at the provider's office due to concerns about increasing fatigue.

   A. According to the theory of Erik Erikson, which life stage would this patient's age fall within?

   ____

   ____

   ____

   B. According to Erik Erikson's stages of psychosocial development, what developmental stage does this age group address?

   ____

   ____

   ____

   C. According to the theory of Erik Erikson, what care considerations should be considered when working with this age group?

   ____

   ____

   ____

© 2017 Cengage Learning. All Rights Reserved. May not be scanned, copied or duplicated, or posted to a publicly accessible website, in whole or in part.

UNIT 4
Personal and Workplace Safety

© 2017 Cengage Learning. All Rights Reserved. May not be scanned, copied or duplicated, or posted to a publicly accessible website, in whole or in part.

CHAPTER 9

Body Mechanics

LEARNING OBJECTIVES

Studying and applying the material in this chapter will help you to:

- Understand and explain the importance of practicing good body mechanics and ergonomics at all times to prevent injury.
- Explain how repetitive injuries occur and how to prevent them.
- Demonstrate proper methods of sitting when working to prevent injury.
- Demonstrate proper methods of walking and standing at work to prevent injury.
- Demonstrate proper methods of lifting to prevent injury.
- Demonstrate proper methods of working at the computer to prevent injury.
- Properly use special adaptive devices to reduce the risk of workplace injuries.

VOCABULARY REVIEW

Definitions

Write the definition of each of the following words or terms.

1. body mechanics

____

____

____

2. ergonomics

____

____

____

© 2017 Cengage Learning. All Rights Reserved. May not be scanned, copied or duplicated, or posted to a publicly accessible website, in whole or in part.

3. repetitive motion injury (RMI)

____

____

____

CHAPTER REVIEW

Identification 1

Place an "X" in front of the factors that can increase the likelihood of injury.

_____ 1. poor posture

_____ 2. poor body mechanics

_____ 3. low level of fitness

_____ 4. obesity

_____ 5. mechanical stress

_____ 6. psychological stress

Identification 2

Place an "X" in front of actions that specify proper sitting habits.

_____ 1. Do not use a chair back.

_____ 2. Keep head and shoulders aligned over hips.

_____ 3. When turning, pivot from the neck.

_____ 4. Position chair so work is slightly below eye level.

_____ 5. Place feet flat on the floor or on a footrest.

Identification 3

Place an "X" in front of actions that specify proper standing or walking.

_____ 1. Keep neck in a neutral position.

_____ 2. When standing, keep weight evenly distributed on both feet at all times.

_____ 3. If possible, take off shoes and wear only socks or go barefoot.

_____ 4. When standing, alternate placing one foot up on a footstool.

_____ 5. Maintain the three normal curves of the back.

© 2017 Cengage Learning. All Rights Reserved. May not be scanned, copied or duplicated, or posted to a publicly accessible website, in whole or in part.

Identification 4

Place an "X" in front of actions that specify proper lifting.

_____ 1. Increase the base of support by positioning feet 12 to 15 inches apart.

_____ 2. Position your hands underneath the object to be lifted.

_____ 3. Exhale before lifting a heavy object.

_____ 4. Carry objects approximately 6 inches from the body at pelvic level.

_____ 5. When turning, move your entire body in unison.

Identification 5

Place an "X" in front of recommendations to help prevent eyestrain.

_____ 1. Keep the computer screen clean.

_____ 2. Rest the eyes every 1 to 2 hours.

_____ 3. Use a glare screen on the computer.

_____ 4. Use a paper holder to prevent having to look down to see text.

_____ 5. Adjust the contrast on the computer screen to a minimal level.

True/False

Indicate whether the following statements are true (T) or false (F).

_____ 1. Injuries are usually the result of poor practices over time that involve the repetition of improper movements.

_____ 2. The greatest number of accidents in health care are the result of one-time incidents.

_____ 3. Aging makes the health care professional more prone to injury.

_____ 4. Most injuries are cumulative, and so it is habitual activity repeated over years that determines the future risk of injury.

_____ 5. Ergonomics is the correct positioning of the body for a given task, such as lifting a heavy object or typing.

_____ 6. RMI refer only to those injuries that are sustained while performing work duties.

_____ 7. When standing in a static position, taking a break every two hours will avoid injury.

_____ 8. Tension reduces blood circulation in the affected tissues and contributes to injury.

_____ 9. Surgical intervention is the most common method of treating RMIs.

_____ 10. Back injuries account for nearly 20% of all injuries and illnesses in the workplace.

_____ 11. People who wear bifocals have an additional challenge to overcome when working on the computer.

© 2017 Cengage Learning. All Rights Reserved. May not be scanned, copied or duplicated, or posted to a publicly accessible website, in whole or in part.

Multiple Choice

Circle the best answer for each of the following questions. There is only one correct answer to each question.

1. Which of the following makes the health care professional more prone to injury?
   A. increased flexibility
   B. decreased flexibility
   C. decreased recovery time
2. Which of the following stressors contribute to work injuries?
   A. mechanical stress
   B. psychological stress
   C. both mechanical and psychological stresses
3. Which of the following is defined as using the correct positioning of the body for a given task?
   A. body mechanics
   B. ergonomics
   C. posture
4. Which systems are most often involved when a health care professional suffers a work injury?
   A. digestive and endocrine
   B. integumentary and sensory
   C. musculoskeletal and nervous
5. Which of the following RMIs is caused by repeated hand motions that pinch a nerve in the wrist?
   A. carpal tunnel syndrome
   B. thoracic outlet syndrome
   C. tendonitis
6. Which of the following RMIs is caused by repeated motions that compress nerves in the neck?
   A. carpal tunnel syndrome
   B. thoracic outlet syndrome
   C. tendonitis
7. Which of the following RMIs is caused by repeated motion in a joint that inflames the tendons?
   A. carpal tunnel syndrome
   B. thoracic outlet syndrome
   C. tendonitis
8. Which of the following is a symptom of tendonitis?
   A. tenderness in the tendons of the shoulders, elbows, or hands
   B. tingling in the face and neck
   C. inability to make a fist
9. Which of the following is a symptom of thoracic outlet syndrome?
   A. inability to make a fist
   B. foot pain
   C. weakness in arms and hands

© 2017 Cengage Learning. All Rights Reserved. May not be scanned, copied or duplicated, or posted to a publicly accessible website, in whole or in part.

10. Which of the following is a symptom of carpal tunnel syndrome?
    A. leg pain
    B. loss of strength in the hand
    C. shoulder pain
11. Which of the following statements is true about the use of a mouse as a pointing device?
    A. It is effective in reducing injuries.
    B. It increases injuries.
    C. It has no impact on the injury rate.

Short Answer

Read each question. Think about the information presented in the text, and then answer each question.

1. What are the common symptoms of RMIs?

   ____

   ____

   ____

2. List five conservative treatment measures for injuries.

   ____

   ____

   ____

3. What impact have computers had on the number of work injuries? List five preventive measures to follow while using a computer.

   ____

   ____

   ____

Critical Thinking Scenarios

Read each scenario. Think about the information presented in the text, and then answer each question.

1. Martha Zamboni is a 55-year-old health care professional. She is exhausted by her demanding schedule and family and social responsibilities. She keeps setting start dates to begin a healthful eating and exercise program. She is 5′5″ tall and weighs 180 pounds.

   A. Is Martha at a higher risk for injury?

      ____

      ____

      ____

© 2017 Cengage Learning. All Rights Reserved. May not be scanned, copied or duplicated, or posted to a publicly accessible website, in whole or in part.

B. What factors put her at risk?

___

___

___

C. What preventive measures could she take to decrease her risk?

___

___

___

2. Peter Phillips is a health care professional whose job requires a lot of lifting and carrying of heavy items. He says he has heard some good things about back belts and asks your opinion.

   A. Should you recommend he wear a back belt?

   ___

   ___

   ___

   B. What are the possible advantages to wearing a back belt?

   ___

   ___

   ___

   C. What are the possible disadvantages to wearing a back belt?

   ___

   ___

   ___

© 2017 Cengage Learning. All Rights Reserved. May not be scanned, copied or duplicated, or posted to a publicly accessible website, in whole or in part.

CHAPTER 10

Infection Control

LEARNING OBJECTIVES

Studying and applying the material in this chapter will help you to:

- Understand and explain the importance of infection control practices in maintaining the safety of the health care professional, patients, and others.
- List the milestones that led to the development of germ theory and infection control.
- Identify the five types of microbes and give examples of infectious diseases caused by each type.
- Describe the chain of infection and list methods the health care professional can use to break it.
- Give examples of the body's defense mechanisms.
- Describe the CDC and OSHA and explain their roles in health care safety.
- Identify the preventive procedures included in the standard precautions.
- Identify situations when handwashing is indicated and demonstrate the technique.
- Identify the three types of transmission-based precautions and when they may be used.
- Describe neutropenic precautions and when they would be used.
- Explain the differences among antiseptics, disinfectants, and sterilization.
- Identify and describe the three major disease risks for health care professionals.
- Describe how pathogens become drug resistant and the impact this has on health care.
- Describe measures that will protect the health care professional and others from blood-borne pathogens.

© 2017 Cengage Learning. All Rights Reserved. May not be scanned, copied or duplicated, or posted to a publicly accessible website, in whole or in part.

VOCABULARY REVIEW

Definitions

Write the definition of each of the following words or terms.

1. aerobic

2. AIDS

3. anaerobic

4. antibiotic

5. antiseptics

6. asepsis (aseptic technique)

7. bacteria

8. bacteriocidal

© 2017 Cengage Learning. All Rights Reserved. May not be scanned, copied or duplicated, or posted to a publicly accessible website, in whole or in part.

9. bacteriostatic

10. Centers for Disease Control and Prevention (CDC)

11. chain of infection

12. communicable disease

13. contaminated

14. disinfectants

15. fungi (pl. of fungus)

© 2017 Cengage Learning. All Rights Reserved. May not be scanned, copied or duplicated, or posted to a publicly accessible website, in whole or in part.

Matching 1

Match the following terms with their correct definitions.

_____	1. germ theory	A.	states that specific microorganisms called bacteria are the cause of specific diseases in both humans and animals
_____	2. hepatitis B	B.	living plants or animals from which microorganisms derive nourishment
_____	3. HIV positive	C.	procedures to decrease the numbers and spread of pathogens in the environment
_____	4. host	D.	scientific study of microorganisms
_____	5. immune response	E.	isolation procedures to protect an immunocompromised patient from infections
_____	6. infection control	F.	infection that occurs while the patient is receiving health care
_____	7. infectious disease	G.	microorganisms that commonly reside in a particular environment on or in the body
_____	8. medical asepsis (clean technique)	H.	instrument fitted with a powerful magnifying lens
_____	9. microbes	I.	small, usually one-celled living plants or animals
_____	10. microbiology	J.	microorganisms that are pathogenic
_____	11. microorganisms	K.	disease caused by growth of pathogens
_____	12. microscope	L.	a virus that causes a blood-borne infection; an occupational hazard for health care workers
_____	13. neutropenic precautions	M.	the condition of being infected by the human immunodeficiency virus
_____	14. normal flora	N.	defense used by the body to fight infection and disease by producing antibodies
_____	15. nosocomial infection	O.	procedures to be followed to prevent the spread of infectious diseases

© 2017 Cengage Learning. All Rights Reserved. May not be scanned, copied or duplicated, or posted to a publicly accessible website, in whole or in part.

Word Fill

Complete the following sentences by filling in the missing words.

opportunistic infection	Occupational Safety and Health Administration	parasite standard precautions	pathogens sterile field
protozoa sterilization viruses	rickettsia surgical asepsis (sterile technique)	transmission-based precautions	tuberculosis (TB)

1. The abbreviation OSHA stands for ______________________.
2. A/An ______________________ is an area designated to be free of microorganisms.
3. ______________________ are infections that occurs due to the weakened physiological state of the body.
4. ______________________ are the smallest of the microbes; they cannot be seen under normal light.
5. ______________________ uses agents or methods that totally destroy all microorganisms, including viruses and spores.
6. A/An ______________________ is an organism that nourishes itself at the expense of other living things and causes them damage.
7. ______________________ are procedures to completely eliminate the presence of pathogens from objects and areas.
8. ______________________ are practices designed to reduce the risk of transmission of microorganisms from both recognized and unrecognized sources of infection in health care settings.
9. A/An ______________________ are disease-causing microorganisms.
10. ______________________ include three types of isolation procedures (airborne, droplet, and contact precautions) required for specific infections.
11. ______________________ is a disease caused by the contagious, airborne pathogen *Mycobacterium tuberculosis*.
12. ______________________ are microorganisms that are classified as animals.
13. ______________________ are microorganisms that are smaller than bacteria and have rod or spherical shapes.

CHAPTER REVIEW

Identification 1

Place an "X" in front of the steps that are part of correct handwashing technique.

_____ 1. Keep hands lower than the elbow.

_____ 2. Scrub palms in a circular motion while clasping hands together.

_____ 3. Scrub wrists and forearms up to the elbows.

_____ 4. Scrub hands for at least 2 minutes.

© 2017 Cengage Learning. All Rights Reserved. May not be scanned, copied or duplicated, or posted to a publicly accessible website, in whole or in part.

_____ 5. Rinse thoroughly with warm running water from the wrists down to the fingertips.

_____ 6. Clean under the nails with a cuticle stick, a brush, a fingernail, or by rubbing it against the palm of the other hand.

_____ 7. Use bar soap and create a good lather.

Identification 2

Place an "X" in front of the items that are considered personal protective equipment (PPE).

_____ 1. masks

_____ 2. glasses/goggles

_____ 3. gowns

_____ 4. caps

_____ 5. dressings

_____ 6. gloves

True/False

Indicate whether the following statements are true (T) or false (F).

_____ 1. Medical asepsis is also known as sterile technique.

_____ 2. The Centers for Disease Control and Prevention (CDC) and the Occupational Safety and Health Administration (OSHA) are both governmental agencies.

_____ 3. Someone with a nosocomial infection should be placed in isolation.

_____ 4. Flagella are whip-like appendages that help certain bacteria move.

_____ 5. Viruses are obligate intracellular organisms.

_____ 6. Normal flora are a common source of infection.

_____ 7. *Escherichia coli* (*E. coli*) can be both pathogenic and nonpathogenic.

_____ 8. An immune response is an abnormal response of the body.

_____ 9. Generalized infections can easily be treated by applying a local antibiotic.

_____ 10. An anaerobic microorganism does not require oxygen to live.

© 2017 Cengage Learning. All Rights Reserved. May not be scanned, copied or duplicated, or posted to a publicly accessible website, in whole or in part.

Matching 2

Match the following terms with their correct definitions.

____ 1.	bacteria	A.	used with infectious organisms that can be propelled short distance through the air
____ 2.	viruses	B.	only microbes that are classified as animals
____ 3.	fungi	C.	used when infectious organisms are transmitted by touching of skin or other surfaces
____ 4.	rickettsia	D.	used for patients very susceptible to infections
____ 5.	protozoa	E.	smaller than bacteria and have rod or spherical shapes
____ 6.	airborne precautions	F.	smallest of the microbes
____ 7.	droplet precautions	G.	one-celled plants
____ 8.	contact precautions	H.	used for patients with diagnosis of *Mycobacterium tuberculosis*
____ 9.	standard precautions	I.	large group of organisms that are neither plant nor animal
____ 10.	neutropenic precautions	J.	must be used at all times to prevent contact with potentially infectious body fluids

Matching 3

Match the following terms with their correct definitions.

____ 1.	avian influenza	A.	transmitted by infected mosquitoes to humans and animals
____ 2.	bovine spongiform encephalopathy	B.	caused by a resistant strain of *Staphylococcus aureus*
____ 3.	West Nile virus	C.	transmitted by infected birds
____ 4.	H1N1 influenza	D.	caused by a resistant strain of enterococci
____ 5.	MRSA	E.	spread mainly person-to-person
____ 6.	VRE	F.	thought to be caused by a type of protein, called prions, normally found in animals

Short Answer

Read each question. Think about the information presented in the text, and then answer each question.

1. List three of the natural defense mechanisms of the body.

____

____

____

© 2017 Cengage Learning. All Rights Reserved. May not be scanned, copied or duplicated, or posted to a publicly accessible website, in whole or in part.

2. What is the difference between medical asepsis and surgical asepsis?

3. How can the health care professional decrease the source of microorganisms?

4. How can the health care professional prevent the transmission of microorganisms?

5. How can the health care professional maximize the resistance of the host?

6. List the various hepatitis viruses and how they are transmitted.

7. What is the difference between being HIV positive and having AIDS?

8. Explain how someone can have a positive TB skin test and not have active tuberculosis.

9. What are the signs and symptoms of active TB disease?

10. Why is it important to immediately report accidental exposures to blood or body fluids to the supervisor?

© 2017 Cengage Learning. All Rights Reserved. May not be scanned, copied or duplicated, or posted to a publicly accessible website, in whole or in part.

Labeling

Assign the labels from the list to the appropriate places on the figure.

Figure 10–1 Chain of Infection

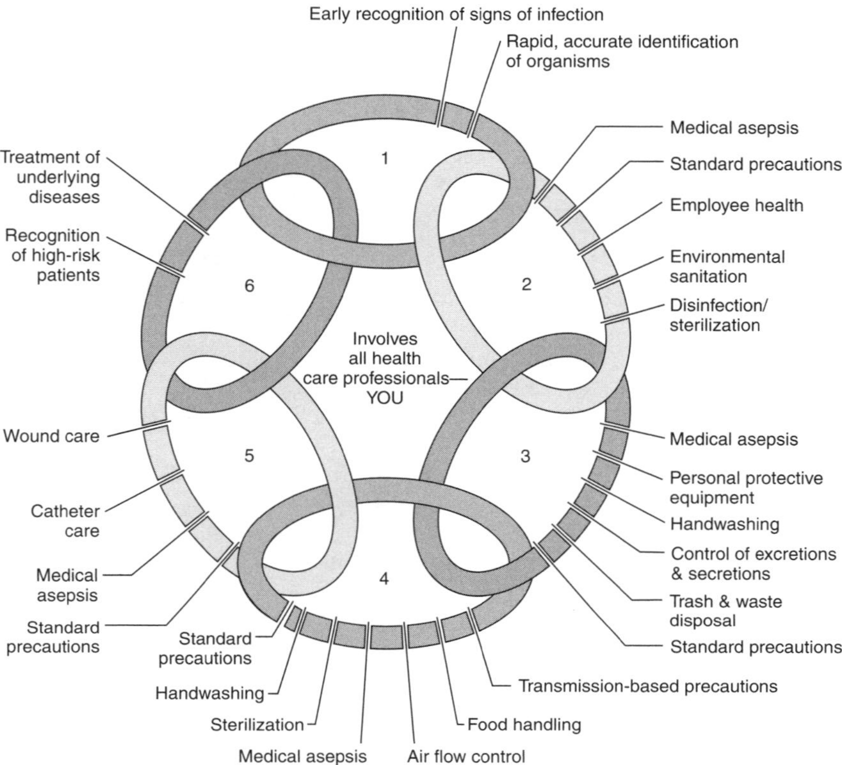

1. _____ susceptible host
2. _____ infectious agent
3. _____ route of transmission
4. _____ portal of entry
5. _____ portal of exit
6. _____ reservoir host

Critical Thinking Scenarios

Read each scenario. Think about the information presented in the text, and then answer each question.

1. Magreet Hawking is very concerned about getting swine flu and has many questions when she comes to the health care facility.

   A. How is H1N1 transmitted?

   ____

   ____

   ____

   B. What are the common symptoms?

   ____

   ____

   ____

© 2017 Cengage Learning. All Rights Reserved. May not be scanned, copied or duplicated, or posted to a publicly accessible website, in whole or in part.

C. What preventive measures can she use?

____

____

____

2. Stephen Quest has been reading about the increase in community-associated MRSA and asks for more information from his health care professional.

   A. What is the difference between HA-MRSA and CA-MRSA?

   ____

   ____

   ____

   B. What has caused the development of resistant bacteria?

   ____

   ____

   ____

   C. What can he do to decrease the chances of contracting a CA-MRSA infection?

   ____

   ____

   ____

   D. How can you as a health care professional help prevent your patients from developing a HA-MRSA?

   ____

   ____

   ____

Procedure Assessments

Complete the procedure assessments for this chapter at the end of the workbook.

© 2017 Cengage Learning. All Rights Reserved. May not be scanned, copied or duplicated, or posted to a publicly accessible website, in whole or in part.

CHAPTER 11

Environmental Safety

LEARNING OBJECTIVES

Studying and applying the material in this chapter will help you to:

- Understand and explain the importance of environmental safety in maintaining the safety of the health care professional, the patients, and others.
- Identify general safety guidelines that will help prevent injuries and accidents in health care facilities.
- Describe and give examples of how changes in the physical and mental health of a patient can increase the risk of injuries and accidents.
- Define what workplace violence is and discuss preventive measures.
- Describe and explain the purpose of an incident report.
- Identify the appropriate steps to take in the event of a fire.
- Identify the different classes of fire extinguishers and type of fire on which to use each.
- List ways to prevent electrical hazards.
- Discuss chemical, radiation, and infectious hazards and the role of the health care professional in their prevention.
- Describe the precautions necessary when oxygen is in use.
- Explain when an emergency preparedness plan would be implemented and define a triage system.

© 2017 Cengage Learning. All Rights Reserved. May not be scanned, copied or duplicated, or posted to a publicly accessible website, in whole or in part.

VOCABULARY

Definitions

Write the definition of each of the following words or terms.

1. compatibility

____

____

____

2. flammable

____

____

____

3. toxic

____

____

____

Matching 1

Match the following terms with their correct definitions.

_____ 1. emergency preparedness plan

_____ 2. environmental safety

_____ 3. incident report

_____ 4. inflammable

_____ 5. PASS

_____ 6. RACE

_____ 7. triage system

A. guidelines to determine which patients to send where and what treatment will be given during an emergency

B. written document that is filled out when any unexpected situation occurs that can cause harm to a patient, employee, or any other person

C. policy and procedures to be followed when an event occurs that has the potential to kill or injure a group of people

D. acronym for responding to fires

E. acronym for proper use of a portable fire extinguisher

F. easily set on fire; same as flammable

G. the identification and correction of potential hazards that can cause accidents and injuries

© 2017 Cengage Learning. All Rights Reserved. May not be scanned, copied or duplicated, or posted to a publicly accessible website, in whole or in part.

CHAPTER REVIEW

True/False

Indicate whether the following statements are true (T) or false (F).

_____ 1. Patients have the right to refuse any procedure or medication.

_____ 2. You can leave a patient unattended on a treatment table if they are alert and oriented.

_____ 3. If a patient is hard of hearing the best approach is to yell very loudly when communicating.

_____ 4. If the patient has tremors or shaking it may be a sign of an altered neurological function.

_____ 5. Patients taking medications should be observed for changes that can affect their safety.

_____ 6. The health care area is a very safe place to work, and health care professionals are rarely exposed to safety and health hazards.

_____ 7. Fires in health care facilities can result from a number of hazards.

_____ 8. It is critical to stay calm during an emergency.

_____ 9. A policy that many facilities have is that no personal electrical equipment can be brought into the hospital because the possibility of it being defective is a fire risk.

_____ 10. When smoke is present during a fire it is best to walk upright as there will be more oxygen at higher levels.

Multiple Choice

Circle the best answer for each of the following questions. There is only one correct answer to each question.

1. When would it be appropriate to run in a health care facility?

   A. in an emergency
   B. during a fire
   C. never

2. Which side of the hallway should be walked on in a health care facility?

   A. right
   B. left
   C. center

3. When is it appropriate to wear earrings in a health care facility?

   A. never
   B. when they do not extend beyond the earlobe
   C. when you are not working with combative patients

4. What is the main reason for keeping fingernails short when working in a health care facility?

   A. prevents scratching of patients
   B. prevents painful tears when they catch on items
   C. they harbor bacteria

© 2017 Cengage Learning. All Rights Reserved. May not be scanned, copied or duplicated, or posted to a publicly accessible website, in whole or in part.

5. What type of jewelry is acceptable in the health care facility?
   A. smooth wedding band
   B. necklaces but not rings or bracelets
   C. no jewelry should be worn
6. How should hair be worn when working in a health care facility?
   A. any style as long as it is kept out of your eyes
   B. tie long hair back or up
   C. place long hair under your collar when bending over patients
7. What type of shoes are to be worn in the health care environment?
   A. only those that have very cushioned soles
   B. any type as long as they are comfortable
   C. enclosed shoes
8. Which of the following ways of identifying patients would be the best?
   A. have them state their name
   B. ask them "Are you ... ?"
   C. have them state their full name and birthdate
9. In what locations is it appropriate to wear your uniform?
   A. only in the work setting
   B. when running an errand right after work
   C. anytime as long as it is clean
10. When should unsafe conditions be reported?
   A. immediately
   B. before the end of your shift
   C. only if you are sure no one else has already made a report

Matching 2

Match the following types of hazards with their descriptions.

_____	1. chemical	A. agents that can cause physical injury and tissue damage
_____	2. environmental	B. unsafe conditions in the workplace
_____	3. ergonomic	C. stressors causing anxiety and emotional fatigue
_____	4. infectious	D. substances with toxic effects when inhaled, ingested, or with skin contact
_____	5. physical	E. microbes that can cause infections
_____	6. psychosocial	F. unsafe workplace design
_____	7. workplace violence	G. physical or verbal abuse

© 2017 Cengage Learning. All Rights Reserved. May not be scanned, copied or duplicated, or posted to a publicly accessible website, in whole or in part.

Short Answer

Read each question. Think about the information presented in the text, and then answer each question.

1. List the various types of fire and which fire extinguishers should be used for each type.

2. Explain what the acronym RACE stands for.

3. Explain what the acronym PASS stands for.

4. What are radiation hazards and how are employees protected?

5. Why are special precautions needed when a patient is receiving oxygen therapy?

6. What is an emergency preparedness plan?

7. What is a triage system?

© 2017 Cengage Learning. All Rights Reserved. May not be scanned, copied or duplicated, or posted to a publicly accessible website, in whole or in part.

Ordering

Place the following duties in the order in which they should be performed when using a fire extinguisher. Put a numeral 1 before the first duty, a 2 before the next, and so on.

_____ sweep back and forth along the base of the fire

_____ pull the pin

_____ aim the nozzle at the base of the fire

_____ squeeze the handle

Labeling

Assign the labels in the list to the appropriate places on the figure.

Figure 11–1

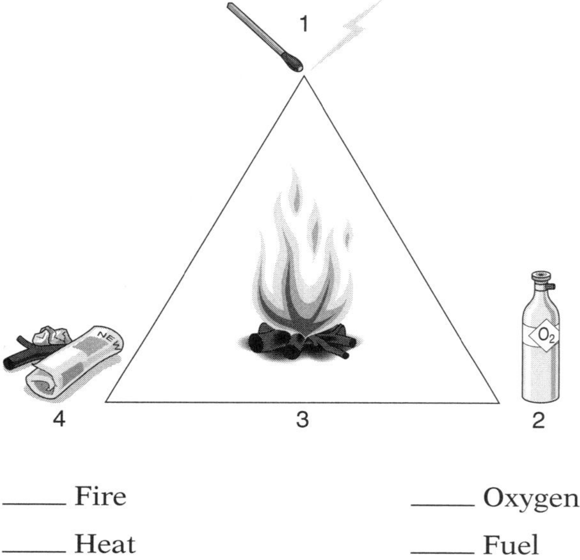

_____ Fire

_____ Heat

_____ Oxygen

_____ Fuel

Assign the labels in the list to the appropriate places on the figure.

Figure 11–2

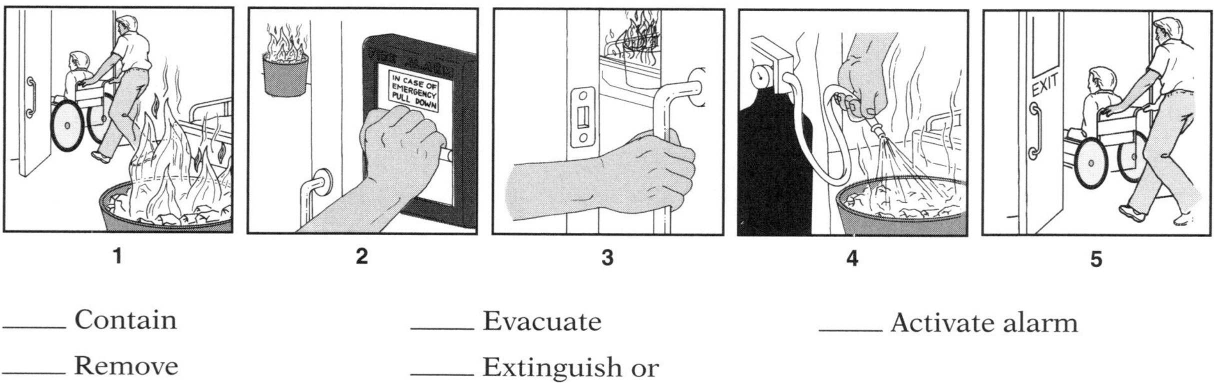

_____ Contain

_____ Remove

_____ Evacuate

_____ Extinguish or

_____ Activate alarm

© 2017 Cengage Learning. All Rights Reserved. May not be scanned, copied or duplicated, or posted to a publicly accessible website, in whole or in part.

Critical Thinking Scenarios

Read each scenario. Think about the information presented in the text, and then answer each question.

1. Mr. Amos Scruthers is concerned about recent articles he has read on bioterrorism and starts to express concern to you while at the health care facility.

   A. Is bioterrorism a new occurrence specific to our current times?

   ___

   ___

   ___

   B. Do health care facilities have any plans in the event of a bioterrorism attack?

   ___

   ___

   ___

   C. What are the most likely threat agents and what precautions would be used?

   ___

   ___

   ___

2. Randy Johnson just accepted a position in the emergency department of a local hospital. He has heard that emergency departments tend to have more workplace violence and is nervous.

   A. What actions constitute workplace violence?

   ___

   ___

   ___

   B. How common is workplace violence?

   ___

   ___

   ___

   C. What is the source of the most common workplace violence?

   ___

   ___

   ___

   D. What can he do to protect himself?

   ___

   ___

   ___

© 2017 Cengage Learning. All Rights Reserved. May not be scanned, copied or duplicated, or posted to a publicly accessible website, in whole or in part.

UNIT 5
Behaviors for Success

© 2017 Cengage Learning. All Rights Reserved. May not be scanned, copied or duplicated, or posted to a publicly accessible website, in whole or in part.

CHAPTER 12

Lifestyle Management

LEARNING OBJECTIVES

Studying and applying the material in this chapter will help you to:

- Explain why it is important for health care professionals to practice a healthy lifestyle.
- List six techniques for developing positive habits.
- List the essential nutrients and the function of each.
- Describe how each of the following contributes to healthy living: diet, physical activity, sleep, and preventive measures.
- Define stress and list several common causes.
- Describe five ways of effectively dealing with stress.
- Explain the major health risks encountered by the health care professional.
- List the causes and symptoms of and preventive measures for burnout.
- Explain how health care professionals can help patients develop good health habits.

VOCABULARY REVIEW

Definitions

Write the definition of each of the following words or terms.

1. assertiveness

____

____

____

2. attitude

____

____

____

© 2017 Cengage Learning. All Rights Reserved. May not be scanned, copied or duplicated, or posted to a publicly accessible website, in whole or in part.

3. meditation

____

____

____

4. prioritize

____

____

____

5. relaxation (muscles)

____

____

____

6. stress

____

____

____

7. stressor

____

____

____

Matching 1

Match the following terms with their correct definitions.

____	1. amino acids	A.	food substances that provide the most concentrated form of energy
____	2. carbohydrates	B.	the basic components of protein
____	3. fats	C.	inorganic substances needed for certain body functions
____	4. fiber	D.	food substances needed for building and maintaining body structures
____	5. minerals	E.	food products that cannot be digested
____	6. proteins	F.	organic substances needed to maintain health
____	7. vitamins	G.	food substances made up of sugar that provide the body with quick energy

© 2017 Cengage Learning. All Rights Reserved. May not be scanned, copied or duplicated, or posted to a publicly accessible website, in whole or in part.

Matching 2

Match the following terms with their correct definitions.

____	1. cholesterol	A.	molecules with unpaired electrons that can damage the body's cells
____	2. diet	B.	a class of plants that includes peas, beans, peanuts, lentils, and soybeans
____	3. free radicals	C.	the process of obtaining food necessary for health and growth
____	4. legumes	D.	the foods a person customarily eats
____	5. nutrients	E.	fatty substances, contained in certain foods, that can accumulate in the arteries
____	6. nutrition	F.	substances the body needs to function and grow
____	7. trans fat	G.	vegetable oil that contains added hydrogen and has the capacity to raise "bad cholesterol" levels in the blood

Word Fill 1

Complete the following sentences by filling in the missing words.

overweight	bulimia	obese	type 2 diabetes
anorexia nervosa	burnout	osteoporosis	binge eating

1. ________________ is a serious physical and psychological disorder characterized by refusing to eat an adequate amount to maintain good health.
2. The practice of compulsively eating large amounts of food, beyond what is needed to satisfy physical hunger, is called ________________.
3. Individuals who make themselves vomit after eating in order to avoid weight gain may be suffering from ________________.
4. Feeling exhausted and unappreciated, along with losing interest in one's job, are signs of ________________.
5. Harold's physician told him he is now ________________, having reaching a BMI of 32.
6. Many older adults have ________________, a condition characterized by bones that have lost their density and are easily fractured.
7. At this time, at least 69% of Americans are either ________________ or obese.
8. ________________ is a serious chronic disease in which blood sugar levels are abnormally high.

© 2017 Cengage Learning. All Rights Reserved. May not be scanned, copied or duplicated, or posted to a publicly accessible website, in whole or in part.

Word Fill 2

Complete the following sentences by filling in the missing words.

metabolism	calories	aerobic	Choose My Plate
organic	body mass index		

1. ________________ exercise increases the strength of the heart muscle.
2. The measurement of the relationship of weight to height using a mathematical formula is called the ________________.
3. ________________ are units of energy from food that the body uses to function or store as fat.
4. The U.S. Department of Agriculture developed ________________ to help individuals plan meals that contain required nutrients.
5. The chemical process of converting nutrients into tissue and/or producing energy is called ________________.
6. When referring to agricultural products, ________________ describes certain production methods that include using natural rather than chemical fertilizers and pesticides.

CHAPTER REVIEW

True/False

Indicate whether the following statements are true (T) or false (F).

_____ 1. Many serious health conditions, such as heart disease, are strongly influenced by lifestyle habits.

_____ 2. Most people with arthritis feel better if they avoid physical exercise.

_____ 3. Physical exercise promotes the body's production of endorphins.

_____ 4. Most people do best when they get about six hours of sleep each night.

_____ 5. It is recommended that adults get at least one hour of physical activity every day.

_____ 6. People who have trouble sleeping may find that avoiding stressful activities in the evening improves their ability to sleep.

_____ 7. Gum disease is usually not serious and can be ignored as long as it isn't painful.

_____ 8. Health care professionals who may contact body fluids as part of their work should be immunized against hepatitis B.

_____ 9. Stress is defined as an emotional reaction to an irritating or annoying event.

_____ 10. A good way to maintain good health is to avoid all stressful situations.

_____ 11. When faced with many responsibilities, it is best to do the easiest tasks first.

_____ 12. Meditating regularly can bring about positive physiological changes.

© 2017 Cengage Learning. All Rights Reserved. May not be scanned, copied or duplicated, or posted to a publicly accessible website, in whole or in part.

True/False Rewrite

Please rewrite the bold part of the sentence to make the statement true.

1. Fiber is needed **only by persons who have digestive problems.**

2. Developing healthy habits **is easy** for individuals with strong willpower and self-discipline.

3. A healthy diet should contain adequate amounts of protein and **no fats.**

4. Foods containing high amounts of **proteins,** such as fish, provide the most concentrated forms of energy.

5. Water makes up about **40%** of the average person's total body weight.

6. Amino acids are important components of **carbohydrates.**

7. A diet to help prevent osteoporosis should include high amounts of **vitamin C.**

8. A gram of fat contains **5 calories.**

© 2017 Cengage Learning. All Rights Reserved. May not be scanned, copied or duplicated, or posted to a publicly accessible website, in whole or in part.

9. **Eggs and cheese** are good sources of omega-3 fatty acids.

____

____

____

10. Approximately **40%** of the adults in the United States are either overweight or obese.

____

____

____

Matching 3

Match the following vitamins with their functions. (Note: Two of the vitamins perform the same function.)

_____ 1. vitamin A	A.	production of energy from carbohydrates
_____ 2. thiamin	B.	manufacture of amino acids and red blood cells
_____ 3. riboflavin	C.	normal function of muscles
_____ 4. niacin	D.	healing of wounds; healthy bones and gums
_____ 5. vitamin B_6	E.	growth; prevention of infection
_____ 6. vitamin B_{12}	F.	absorption of calcium
_____ 7. vitamin C	G.	metabolism of nutrients into energy
_____ 8. vitamin D	H.	clotting of blood
_____ 9. vitamin E	I.	production of red blood cells; maintenance of nervous system
_____ 10. vitamin K		

Matching 4

Match the following minerals with their functions.

_____ 1. calcium	A.	nerve function; muscle contraction
_____ 2. folate	B.	transport of oxygen in red blood cells
_____ 3. iron	C.	growth and repair of supportive tissue
_____ 4. magnesium	D.	DNA synthesis in making protein
_____ 5. phosphorus	E.	energy production; nerve function
_____ 6. potassium	F.	reproduction of cells; tissue growth and repair
_____ 7. zinc	G.	building and maintenance of bones

© 2017 Cengage Learning. All Rights Reserved. May not be scanned, copied or duplicated, or posted to a publicly accessible website, in whole or in part.

Short Answer

Read each question. Think about the information presented in the text, and then answer each question.

1. List four factors that contribute to the growing problem of substance abuse among health care professionals.

2. Why it is difficult for many individuals to give up smoking?

3. What is the difference between internal and external stressors?

4. How does relaxing the muscles help relieve feelings of anxiety?

5. What are five positive effects of meditation when it is practiced over an extended period of time?

6. What are four ways that individuals can protect themselves against sexually transmitted diseases?

7. List six occupational stressors that can lead to burnout.

8. List at least six conditions and diseases related to overweight and obesity.

© 2017 Cengage Learning. All Rights Reserved. May not be scanned, copied or duplicated, or posted to a publicly accessible website, in whole or in part.

9. List five methods that have been found helpful for individuals who want to quit smoking.

____

____

____

10. What is the formula for calculating body mass index?

____

____

____

Completion

Use the words in the list to complete the following statements:

high quality	nutrients	reasonable	responsibility
addictive substances	energy	role models	sleep
progress	arthritis		

1. Some habits, such as smoking, are difficult to change because they involve __________.
2. When working to achieve goals, it can be helpful to track your __________ on a chart.
3. Good health is about more than living a long time; it is also about living a __________ life.
4. Medical science can help solve many problems, but individuals must take __________ for their own health.
5. Today's health care professionals should serve as __________ for their patients and for society as a whole.
6. When working to change lifestyle habits, it is best to set __________ goals.
7. Muscle tissue uses more __________ to support itself than does fat tissue.
8. When choosing an eating plan to lose weight, it is important to make sure that all essential __________ are included.
9. One of the many benefits of physical exercise is that it can decrease the pain of __________.
10. Body temperature decreases and functions slow down during __________.

© 2017 Cengage Learning. All Rights Reserved. May not be scanned, copied or duplicated, or posted to a publicly accessible website, in whole or in part.

Critical Thinking Scenarios

Read each scenario. Think about the information presented in the text, and then answer each question.

1. Janna is a practical nurse. She has been working at a nursing home for the last three years. There has been a lot of turnover among staff and she is frequently asked to work extra hours. Many of the residents are elderly and die within months of being admitted. Janna is becoming increasingly unhappy with her job.

   A. What is the name of the condition that Janna may be experiencing?

   ____

   ____

   ____

   B. What are signs of this condition?

   ____

   ____

   ____

   C. What can Janna do to counteract this condition?

   ____

   ____

   ____

2. Earl has a part-time job in addition to his respiratory therapy classes. After studying in the evenings, he finds he is "wound up" and likes to relax by watching television until rather late. Recently, he has found it difficult to concentrate during lectures and when doing his reading assignments.

   A. Explain how Earl's late nights may be contributing to his difficulty concentrating.

   ____

   ____

   ____

   B. When does mental recuperation take place during sleep?

   ____

   ____

   ____

   C. What are some methods Earl might use to increase the quality and quantity of sleep?

   ____

   ____

   ____

© 2017 Cengage Learning. All Rights Reserved. May not be scanned, copied or duplicated, or posted to a publicly accessible website, in whole or in part.

CHAPTER 13

Professionalism

LEARNING OBJECTIVES

Studying and applying the material in this chapter will help you to:

- Explain the meaning of professionalism for individuals who work in health care.
- Describe each of the following components of professionalism:
  - Attitude
  - Behaviors
  - Health care skills
  - Appearance
- Explain the meaning of "professional distance."
- Explain how health care professionals can effectively handle difficult situations.
- Describe how to accept criticism professionally.
- Explain how professional organizations help individuals who work in health care increase their level of professionalism.
- Identify the characteristics of a health care leader.

VOCABULARY REVIEW

Definitions

Write the definition of each of the following words or terms.

1. continuing education

____

____

____

© 2017 Cengage Learning. All Rights Reserved. May not be scanned, copied or duplicated, or posted to a publicly accessible website, in whole or in part.

2. leadership

____

____

____

3. objective (adjective)

____

____

____

4. professional distance

____

____

____

5. professionalism

____

____

____

CHAPTER REVIEW

True/False

Indicate whether the following statements are true (T) or false (F).

_____ 1. Pain and fear can cause patients to behave rudely.

_____ 2. It is inappropriate for a supervisor to ask an employee to do extra work that is not part of the employee's job description.

_____ 3. It is a good idea to get your coworkers' opinions about how to handle problems you are having with your supervisor.

_____ 4. Even experienced health care professionals need to pay attention and think about what they are doing at work.

_____ 5. It is appropriate to ask your supervisor about what to do in a situation with a patient that does not seem right given the circumstances.

_____ 6. The appearance of health professionals is not important as long as they are competent.

_____ 7. Health care professionals should not seek the friendship and approval of their patients.

_____ 8. Understanding the theories that support your skills is not important if you can perform the skills accurately and safely.

_____ 9. Most health care professional organizations try not to get involved with politics at any level.

_____ 10. Good leaders do not necessarily have supervisory positions.

© 2017 Cengage Learning. All Rights Reserved. May not be scanned, copied or duplicated, or posted to a publicly accessible website, in whole or in part.

Multiple Choice

Circle the best answer for each of the following questions. There is only one correct answer to each question.

1. Maintaining professional distance means ________________.

   A. not invading a patient's personal space
   B. not becoming emotionally involved with patients
   C. taking care not to spread infections from one patient to another

2. Kim often has her feelings hurt when patients are not appreciative of her efforts to help them. She should ________________.

   A. ask her supervisor for help with this problem
   B. let her patients know they have hurt her feelings
   C. explore why she feels the need for approval

3. When encountering a difficult situation on the job, it is recommended that health care professionals ________________.

   A. ignore the situation and continue with their work
   B. apply the five-step problem-solving process
   C. ask their supervisor to take care of the problem

4. Larry's supervisor criticized his technique in delivering a breathing treatment. The best course of action for Larry is to ________________.

   A. ask his supervisor for help in perfecting his technique
   B. tell his supervisor that this is how he learned the technique in school
   C. ignore the criticism

5. When patients complain to Gayle, a dietetic technician, about the diets their doctors have prescribed, she should ________________.

   A. say that she is just following the doctor's orders
   B. tell them it's okay for them to "cheat" a little
   C. explain how the diet will improve their health

6. Which of the following best demonstrates the meaning of leadership?

   A. receiving a promotion at work
   B. inspiring coworkers to meet team goals
   C. volunteering to work extra hours

7. Being committed to your work is best demonstrated by ________________.

   A. always putting the needs of patients before your own
   B. believing in the value of your work with patients
   C. developing emotional attachments with your patients

8. The most effective approach to problems in the workplace is ________________.

   A. objective
   B. subjective
   C. biased

9. Tishia, a dental hygienist, is experiencing serious personal problems. It would be best for her to ________________.

   A. let off steam by discussing her problems with coworkers
   B. share them with her favorite patients
   C. keep them to herself while she is at work

© 2017 Cengage Learning. All Rights Reserved. May not be scanned, copied or duplicated, or posted to a publicly accessible website, in whole or in part.

10. If you are unsure about a policy at your workplace, it is best to first ______________.
    A. check the employee manual
    B. ask your supervisor
    C. ask a coworker

Short Answer

Read each question. Think about the information presented in the text, and then answer each question.

1. List eight behaviors that demonstrate professional conduct.

____

____

____

2. What are five characteristics of a professional attitude?

____

____

____

3. What are five characteristics of professional hygiene and appearance?

____

____

____

4. What benefits can health care professionals receive when they are active in their professional organizations?

____

____

____

5. Why is it important for the health care professional to be well organized?

____

____

____

6. What are possible consequences of health care professionals complaining to coworkers and patients about their jobs?

____

____

____

7. How can problems in the workplace be viewed as opportunities?

____

____

____

© 2017 Cengage Learning. All Rights Reserved. May not be scanned, copied or duplicated, or posted to a publicly accessible website, in whole or in part.

8. Why is it important to understand the theories that support your technical skills?

____

____

____

9. Explain the possible effects of a health care professional's appearance and hygiene on patients.

____

____

____

10. Why is it important for health care professionals to remain calm in emergency situations?

____

____

____

Completion

Use the words in the list to complete the following statements:

self-discipline	flexible	malpractice lawsuits	patient welfare
personal problems	caring competence	objective	dependability
patient satisfaction	attitude		

1. Professionalism in health care can be described as _______________.
2. Approaching work positively is a sign of a good _______________.
3. The primary focus of a good health care professional should be _______________.
4. Taking a/an _______________ approach to a situation means basing decisions on facts rather than emotions and opinions.
5. The conduct of individual health care professionals influences _______________ with the facility in which the professionals work.
6. When patients feel they have received poor service, even if treatment outcomes are positive, they are more likely to file _______________.
7. Knowing you can depend on yourself to complete your tasks is a sign of ___________.
8. Health care professionals who follow through and complete their tasks are demonstrating _______________.
9. It is necessary for health care professionals to be _______________ because health care is constantly changing.
10. Health care professionals should never discuss _______________ with their patients.

© 2017 Cengage Learning. All Rights Reserved. May not be scanned, copied or duplicated, or posted to a publicly accessible website, in whole or in part.

Critical Thinking Scenarios

Read each scenario. Think about the information presented in the text, and then answer each question.

1. Cindy is starting her first job since graduating as a veterinary technician. She studied hard throughout her program but realizes that there are additional skills she needs to learn and master.

   A. Why is it important for Cindy to continue to work on her technical skills after graduation?

   ____

   ____

   ____

   B. What can she do to further develop her skills?

   ____

   ____

   ____

2. Brad enjoys his work as a paramedic but was told by his supervisor that he needs to be "more professional" when on the job.

   A. How should Brad respond to his supervisor's comment?

   ____

   ____

   ____

   B. How should health care professionals behave when responding to emergencies?

   ____

   ____

   ____

© 2017 Cengage Learning. All Rights Reserved. May not be scanned, copied or duplicated, or posted to a publicly accessible website, in whole or in part.

CHAPTER 14

Lifelong Learning

LEARNING OBJECTIVES

Studying and applying the material in this chapter will help you to:

- Understand and explain the importance of lifelong learning for the health care professional.
- List the reasons for participating in continuing education opportunities.
- Describe ways you can earn continuing education credits.
- List ways you can incorporate self-directed learning into your everyday life.
- Create a personal plan for self-directed learning.

VOCABULARY REVIEW

Definitions

Write the definition of each of the following words or terms.

1. continuing education units

 ____

 ____

 ____

2. continuing professional education

 ____

 ____

 ____

3. demographics

 ____

 ____

 ____

© 2017 Cengage Learning. All Rights Reserved. May not be scanned, copied or duplicated, or posted to a publicly accessible website, in whole or in part.

4. lifelong learning

____

____

____

5. self-directed learning

____

____

____

CHAPTER REVIEW

Matching

Match the following changes with corresponding learning activities for health care professionals.

____ 1. people are living longer

____ 2. hospital stays are shorter

____ 3. increased ethnic diversity among patients

____ 4. growing interest in complementary medicine

____ 5. more third-party payers

____ 6. emphasis on wellness and patient responsibility

____ 7. heavy use of computers in the workplace

____ 8. incidences of hepatitis and other communicable diseases

____ 9. expanded roles for health care professionals

____ 10. passage of the Patient Protection and Affordable Care Act

____ 11. increasingly sophisticated equipment

____ 12. new diagnostic procedures and treatments

A. acquire skills beyond those specific to one's profession

B. read about treatments such as acupuncture and meditation

C. observe the use of new imaging machines

D. learn to use new software programs

E. study the needs of older adults

F. learn about insurance requirements

G. educate patients who previously could not afford health care

H. learn about the cultural groups that make up your patient population

I. learn and practice standard precautions

J. participate in vendor demonstrations of new equipment

K. learn about healthy lifestyle practices

L. develop skill at delivering patient education on self-care practices

© 2017 Cengage Learning. All Rights Reserved. May not be scanned, copied or duplicated, or posted to a publicly accessible website, in whole or in part.

True/False

Indicate whether the following statements are true (T) or false (F).

_____ 1. Technology is changing faster today than at any time in history.

_____ 2. Health care graduates must continue to learn throughout their careers.

_____ 3. As a result of changes in health care, many professionals are performing a more limited set of tasks.

_____ 4. Most certifying bodies require the completion of certain numbers of continuing education credits to renew professional certification.

_____ 5. One unit of continuing education credit typically requires 30 minutes of class attendance.

_____ 6. The school from which you graduated determines the number of continuing education units you will need to maintain your professional certification.

_____ 7. Most certifying bodies require that proof of professional education be retained for at least ten years.

_____ 8. Online courses are not generally accepted for continuing education credit.

Short Answer

Read each question. Think about the information presented in the text, and then answer each question.

1. List five ways to earn continuing education units.

____

____

____

2. What are five criteria for choosing useful, high quality continuing education?

____

____

____

3. Describe four self-directed learning activities in which a health care professional might engage.

____

____

____

4. List six reliable health information websites.

____

____

____

____

© 2017 Cengage Learning. All Rights Reserved. May not be scanned, copied or duplicated, or posted to a publicly accessible website, in whole or in part.

Completion

Use the words in the list to complete the following statements:

continuing education units	certification	demographics	continuing professional education
traditional duties	lifelong learning	certifying body	self-directed learning

1. __________________ refers to what we do throughout our lives to acquire new information and skills.
2. Studies that monitor shifts in population and record statistics are known as __________________.
3. Most health care professionals are required to earn __________________ in order to keep their certifications current.
4. __________________ is the term for the education that follows graduation and keeps a health professional up-to-date in his or her field.
5. __________________ refers to activities that you plan to acquire new information and skills on your own.
6. Providing documentation of learning beyond one's formal training is necessary to retain one's professional __________________.
7. Many health care professionals are being required to learn to perform more than their __________________.
8. Be sure that any educational activity you engage in to earn continuing education units is approved by the __________________ that requires the units.

Critical Thinking Scenarios

Read each scenario. Think about the information presented in the text, and then answer each question.

1. Brett recently graduated from a nursing program, passed his exams to become a registered nurse, and is working in the emergency department at a big-city hospital in his hometown.

   A. Which recent changes in society and health care are most likely to affect his career as a nurse?

   ____

   ____

   ____

   B. What can Brett do throughout his career to keep current and respond to these changes?

   ____

   ____

   ____

© 2017 Cengage Learning. All Rights Reserved. May not be scanned, copied or duplicated, or posted to a publicly accessible website, in whole or in part.

2. Sanjay is a radiographer. His wife recently returned to school and he is taking over more of the household duties and childcare responsibilities for the couple's three children.

   A. How can Sanjay ensure that, in spite of his busy schedule, he acquires the necessary units for maintaining his state license?

   ____

   ____

   ____

   B. What are some efficient ways that Sanjay can earn the continuing education units needed to maintain his license?

   ____

   ____

   ____

© 2017 Cengage Learning. All Rights Reserved. May not be scanned, copied or duplicated, or posted to a publicly accessible website, in whole or in part.

UNIT 6
Communication in the Health Care Setting

© 2017 Cengage Learning. All Rights Reserved. May not be scanned, copied or duplicated, or posted to a publicly accessible website, in whole or in part.

CHAPTER 15

The Patient as an Individual

LEARNING OBJECTIVES

Studying and applying the material in this chapter will help you to:

- Explain the meaning of the philosophy of individual worth and how it applies to work in health care.
- Define *culture* and describe how it influences all aspects of human beliefs and behavior.
- Give examples of how different cultural groups approach issues of health.
- Describe how to determine the effect of cultural influences on the needs of patients.
- List the five levels of Maslow's hierarchy of needs and give an example of each.
- Recognize common defense mechanisms encountered in health care situations.
- Explain how the health care professional can help patients deal with the experience of loss.

VOCABULARY REVIEW

Matching 1

Match the following terms with their correct definitions.

_____	1. defense mechanism	A.	the belief that every human being has value
_____	2. Maslow's hierarchy of needs	B.	a person's view of himself or herself
_____	3. philosophy of individual worth	C.	unconscious psychological responses to threatening or uncomfortable situations
_____	4. physiological needs	D.	a high-level human need to achieve one's potential
_____	5. self-actualization	E.	a visual representation that ranks human needs
_____	6. self-esteem	F.	physical requirements for maintaining life

© 2017 Cengage Learning. All Rights Reserved. May not be scanned, copied or duplicated, or posted to a publicly accessible website, in whole or in part.

Word Fill

Complete the following sentences by filling in the missing words.

personal space prejudice dominant culture culture

1. ________________ is the term that means the values, shared beliefs, and customs of a group of people.
2. The fundamental beliefs about what most people consider to be ideal behavior make up a society's ________________.
3. The appropriate distance considered appropriate for carrying on a conversation is known as ________________.
4. If John has negative feelings about a classmate simply because she belongs to a certain ethnic group, John is demonstrating ________________.

CHAPTER REVIEW

True/False

Indicate whether the following statements are true (T) or false (F).

_____ 1. It is not necessary to show special consideration to patients who are rude and uncooperative.

_____ 2. Almost everyone has prejudices of some kind.

_____ 3. It is not necessary to agree with the cultural beliefs of patients about health.

_____ 4. It is a waste of time to learn about the health care beliefs of your patients, because they will be treated with the best that Western medicine has to offer.

_____ 5. If you explain self-care procedures carefully, patients will understand and follow your instructions.

_____ 6. Most cultures today respect the importance of being on time and using time efficiently.

_____ 7. In some cultures, it is considered rude not to inquire about one's family.

_____ 8. In the United States, the appropriate distance between two people who are conversing is about 3 feet.

_____ 9. It is best not to assume that just because a person speaks some English, he or she will understand everything you say.

_____ 10. Most cultures consider illness to be physically based.

_____ 11. Religious and spiritual beliefs influence the health care beliefs of many people in the United States.

_____ 12. It is reported that about 60% of people in the United States use prayer to assist them with healing.

_____ 13. *Humors* are body fluids that the members of some cultures believe control the health of the body.

© 2017 Cengage Learning. All Rights Reserved. May not be scanned, copied or duplicated, or posted to a publicly accessible website, in whole or in part.

_____ 14. Because they are natural, herbs are much safer to use for medicinal purposes than pharmaceutical drugs.

_____ 15. Natural, plant-based remedies are not regulated by the Food and Drug Administration.

Matching 2

Match the following defense mechanisms with their correct definitions.

_____	1. compensation	A.	retaining unpleasant thoughts and memories subconsciously
_____	2. control	B.	faking illness to avoid something
_____	3. denial	C.	taking charge in an inappropriate situation when unable to do so in another
_____	4. displacement	D.	redirecting strong feelings about one person to someone else
_____	5. malingering	E.	demonstrating behaviors inappropriate for one's age
_____	6. projection	F.	offering an acceptable, but untrue, reason for one's behavior
_____	7. rationalization	G.	shutting off contact with others
_____	8. regression	H.	placing blame for one's own weaknesses onto someone else
_____	9. repression	I.	doing something unsuitable in an attempt to meet a need
_____	10. withdrawal	J.	pretending that something unpleasant is not true

Short Answer

Read each question. Think about the information presented in the text, and then answer each question.

1. What are three major factors that influence the beliefs and habits of an individual?

____

____

____

____

2. What are five appropriate questions to ask patients about their health care beliefs?

____

____

____

____

© 2017 Cengage Learning. All Rights Reserved. May not be scanned, copied or duplicated, or posted to a publicly accessible website, in whole or in part.

3. What are five examples of beliefs about the source of good health?

4. List nine different beliefs about the cause of illness.

5. What are the five levels of needs proposed by Maslow? List them in order, beginning with the lowest, most basic level.

6. What are five common ways that individuals deal with loss, such as a serious health problem or the death of a spouse?

7. What are four ways that health care professionals can help patients who appear to be demonstrating defense mechanisms feel less threatened?

8. What are five ways that health care professionals can help patients preserve or increase their self-esteem?

© 2017 Cengage Learning. All Rights Reserved. May not be scanned, copied or duplicated, or posted to a publicly accessible website, in whole or in part.

9. Explain how the concept of time differs between various cultural groups.

____

____

____

____

10. What is the meaning of *personal space*?

____

____

____

____

Completion

Use the words in the list to complete the following statements:

direct eye contact	faith healing	yin and yang	the soul
acupuncture	prejudice	stress	
t'ai chi	personal space	philosophy of human worth	

1. The concept that every human being has value and should be treated with respect is called the __________.
2. Drawing a conclusion about a person because he belongs to a certain ethnic group is an example of __________.
3. __________, a series of movements originally developed for self-defense, has health benefits that include improved flexibility and balance.
4. An important concept in Chinese medicine is that illness occurs when __________ is/are out of balance.
5. Controlling the flow of body energy by inserting tiny needles into the skin is called __________.
6. Standing too close to another person when speaking shows a lack of understanding of the concept of __________.
7. In some cultures, touching the head is distressing because it is the location of __________.
8. __________ is a sign of aggression in some cultures and a lack of respect in others.
9. __________ is based on the belief that illness can be cured by prayer and strong religious beliefs.
10. Practitioners of traditional Western medicine are recognizing the close connection of the mind and body, especially the effects of __________ on the body.

© 2017 Cengage Learning. All Rights Reserved. May not be scanned, copied or duplicated, or posted to a publicly accessible website, in whole or in part.

Critical Thinking Scenarios

Read each scenario. Think about the information presented in the text, and then answer each question.

1. James Dixon has called Dr. Adler's office a number of times in the last couple of months complaining of various symptoms. Dr. Adler always sees James and has noted that each time the symptoms are different. To date, he cannot identify what might be causing this variety of symptoms. James always asks Dr. Adler to write an excuse for his employer and on his last visit, he mentioned to the doctor that, "It doesn't really matter if I show up or not, my supervisor hates me."

   A. What are two defense mechanisms that James may be displaying?

   ____

   ____

   ____

   B. How do defense mechanisms help individuals deal with difficult situations?

   ____

   ____

   ____

   C. How might defense mechanisms be helping James deal with his work situation?

   ____

   ____

   ____

2. Claire Mason is an 88-year-old woman who recently entered a long-term care facility. Her family does not live in the area and she is feeling sad and depressed.

   A. What are possible reasons for Claire's feelings of sadness and depression?

   ____

   ____

   ____

   B. How can the nurses in the facility help Claire meet her needs for love and affection?

   ____

   ____

   ____

© 2017 Cengage Learning. All Rights Reserved. May not be scanned, copied or duplicated, or posted to a publicly accessible website, in whole or in part.

CHAPTER 16

The Communication Process

LEARNING OBJECTIVES

Studying and applying the material in this chapter will help you to:

- Explain the importance of effective communication in health care.
- Describe the relationship between effective communication and patient well-being.
- List and describe the six steps of the communication process.
- Define and explain the use of the four types of questions.
- Explain the meaning of nonverbal communication and give examples of three types.
- Explain the meaning of *active listening*.
- Define *empathy* and explain its application in health care.
- Explain the meaning of *feedback* and how it is used in communication.
- Recognize common barriers that can prevent effective communication.
- List the techniques to use when communicating with patients who have special needs.
- Demonstrate professional telephone techniques and explain why it is important to apply them in the health care facility.
- Describe the elements that make up effective patient education.
- List strategies for preparing and giving presentations to groups.
- List three ways to handle situations that involve gossip.

© 2017 Cengage Learning. All Rights Reserved. May not be scanned, copied or duplicated, or posted to a publicly accessible website, in whole or in part.

VOCABULARY REVIEW

Definitions

Write the definition of each of the following words or terms.

1. empathy

____
____
____

2. feedback

____
____
____

3. learning objectives

____
____
____

4. sympathy

____
____
____

Matching 1

Match the following terms with their correct definitions.

____	1. closed-ended	A.	feedback technique to request additional information to illustrate the speaker's meaning
____	2. leading	B.	type of question that includes part of the answer
____	3. open-ended	C.	feedback technique in which listeners state what they hear in their own words
____	4. paraphrasing	D.	type of question that can be answered with one word
____	5. probing	E.	type of question that asks for additional information or clarification
____	6. reflecting	F.	type of question that must be answered with more than a one-word response
____	7. requesting examples	G.	feedback technique that prompts speakers to complete or add information to their original messages

© 2017 Cengage Learning. All Rights Reserved. May not be scanned, copied or duplicated, or posted to a publicly accessible website, in whole or in part.

Word Fill

Complete the following sentences by filling in the missing words.

barriers	nonverbal communication	receiver	communication
pantomime	therapeutic communication	active listening	sender

1. ____________________ is characterized by focusing your full attention on what a speaker is saying.
2. ____________________ that block communication include conditions such as noise and hearing impairments.
3. The process of sending and receiving messages is called ____________________.
4. Information exchanged without the use of words involves ____________________.
5. ____________________ can be an effective way of conveying meaning through acting out and gestures with patients who do not understand English.
6. Another word for the listener in a communication exchange is the ____________________.
7. The ____________________ is the person communicating a message.
8. ____________________ focuses on the learning about the needs of patients and how to best help them.

CHAPTER REVIEW

True/False

Indicate whether the following statements are true (T) or false (F).

_____ 1. The ability to communicate well is as important as having good technical skills.

_____ 2. Using casual words and phrases, such as "you know," is a good way to put patients at ease.

_____ 3. If a patient hesitates briefly when answering a question, it is recommended that the health care professional help by suggesting answers.

_____ 4. Humor is usually not appropriate with patients who are ill or injured.

_____ 5. Many patients who cannot speak and appear unresponsive can hear and experience touch.

_____ 6. Nonverbal communication conveys about 70% of the meaning of a spoken message and may even contradict what is said.

_____ 7. Greeting patients with endearments such as "dear" and "sweetie" is a good way to make them feel comfortable.

_____ 8. Feeling and expressing sympathy is a good way for the health care professional to better understand a patient.

_____ 9. The meaning of gestures varies among cultural groups so they must be used with care.

© 2017 Cengage Learning. All Rights Reserved. May not be scanned, copied or duplicated, or posted to a publicly accessible website, in whole or in part.

_____ 10. The ability to listen is as important for health care professionals as the ability to explain clearly.

_____ 11. Periods of silence during communication are uncomfortable for both parties and should be avoided.

_____ 12. Patients who are facing death generally prefer to be left alone.

_____ 13. Nearly half of all adults age 75 and older have some form of hearing impairment.

_____ 14. When faced with an angry patient, it is recommended that the health care professional start by asking the individual to calm down.

_____ 15. Speaking loudly is not generally helpful when speaking to someone who has a hearing impairment or does not understand English well.

_____ 16. Confidential information regarding health matters can never be left for patients on their telephone answering machines.

_____ 17. Planning ahead and organizing what you are going to say is really necessary only when addressing large groups of people.

_____ 18. It is acceptable to gossip about others if they are not present and there is no chance they will hear what you have said.

_____ 19. Patient information should never be discussed during social conversations.

_____ 20. Most patients do not mind if health care professionals discuss their condition within hearing distance of the patient.

Matching 2

Match the following terms with the examples that best illustrate them.

_____	1. closed-ended	A.	Can you tell me more about when you experience this pain?
_____	2. open-ended	B.	What is your age?
_____	3. probing	C.	What kinds of foods seem to make your heartburn worse?
_____	4. leading	D.	Does your tooth hurt most when you are eating something cold?
_____	5. paraphrasing	E.	I'd like to listen so I can understand how you're feeling about this.
_____	6. reflecting	F.	Am I hearing you say that the medicine doesn't seem to be helping?
_____	7. requesting example	G.	I'm really not comfortable talking about Roy when he's not there.
_____	8. empathy	H.	When we are finished, you will be able to dress the wound properly.
_____	9. learning objective	I.	What are your plans for the future?
_____	10. response to gossip	J.	You told me you've been taking this medication for your diabetes for …

© 2017 Cengage Learning. All Rights Reserved. May not be scanned, copied or duplicated, or posted to a publicly accessible website, in whole or in part.

Short Answer

Read each question. Think about the information presented in the text, and then answer each question.

1. What are four trends in the delivery of health care that have increased the need for good communication skills?

2. How does good communication on the part of the health care professional influence patient well-being?

3. List the six steps in the communication process.

4. What are five factors the health care professional should consider to determine a patient's level of understanding when planning communication goals?

5. Give five organizational strategies you can use when creating long messages so they are easy for the listener to follow.

6. Give six examples of positive body language that may encourage patients to share information.

7. State the pros and cons of using touch with patients.

© 2017 Cengage Learning. All Rights Reserved. May not be scanned, copied or duplicated, or posted to a publicly accessible website, in whole or in part.

8. What are eight characteristics of good listening skills?

___

___

___

9. List five examples of communication barriers commonly encountered in health care settings.

___

___

___

10. What are five examples of actions you can take to more effectively communicate with patients who are in pain?

___

___

___

11. What are five examples of techniques to use when communicating with individuals who have hearing impairments?

___

___

___

12. What are five examples of techniques to use when communicating with individuals who have visual impairments?

___

___

___

13. Why is good telephone technique important in the health care setting?

___

___

___

Ordering

Place the following steps for delivering patient education in the order in which they should be performed. Put a numeral 1 before the first step, a 2 before the next, and so on.

____ Listen.

____ Create the instructional message.

____ Set educational goals.

____ Deliver the instruction.

____ Evaluate.

____ Check for understanding.

© 2017 Cengage Learning. All Rights Reserved. May not be scanned, copied or duplicated, or posted to a publicly accessible website, in whole or in part.

Completion

Use the words in the list to complete the following statements:

telephone	nonverbal communication	hearing impairments	disoriented
barriers	smile	active listening	needs
gossip	patient education		

1. Physical distractions and sensory impairments can present ______________ to communication.
2. The first contact that many patients have with a health care facility is by ______________.
3. Focusing on what another person is saying is a characteristic of ______________
4. Eye contact and leaning toward the speaker are examples of ______________.
5. Proper nutrition and back strengthening exercises are examples of topics for ______________.
6. ______________ has no purpose and should not be allowed in the health care workplace.
7. Make sure there is a light source on your face when speaking with patients who have ______________.
8. Identify yourself and say the patient's name when you are communicating with a patient who is ______________.
9. When speaking to a group about a health topic, plan ahead and identify the ______________ of the audience.
10. A/an ______________ is a universal sign of good will.

Critical Thinking Scenarios

Read each scenario. Think about the information presented in the text, and then answer each question.

1. Carla works at the front desk of a busy urgent care clinic. Her job is to answer the phones and greet patients, learning enough about each to determine in what order they should see the physicians.

   A. What can Carla do to make patients, who sometimes have to wait for her attention, feel welcome and attended to?

   ____

   ____

   ____

   B. What are guidelines she can follow to ensure that her telephone manner is welcoming and professional and that her speech is easy to understand?

   ____

   ____

   ____

© 2017 Cengage Learning. All Rights Reserved. May not be scanned, copied or duplicated, or posted to a publicly accessible website, in whole or in part.

2. Jorge is the clinical medical assistant for a plastic surgeon who performs many in-office procedures. Part of his job is to provide pre- and postoperative patient education.

   A. How does patient education influence patient recovery from surgery?

   ____

   ____

   ____

   B. What should Jorge's first step be when delivering patient education?

   ____

   ____

   ____

   C. How can he check to ensure that a patient has understood his instructions?

   ____

   ____

   ____

3. Ashley works in a skilled nursing facility. She enjoys interacting with the older patients but is finding it challenging to interact with those who have Alzheimer's disease.

   A. What should Ashley do when an Alzheimer's patient exhibits difficult behavior, such shouting and hitting?

   ____

   ____

   ____

   B. What are some strategies she can use to improve her communication with these patients?

   ____

   ____

   ____

© 2017 Cengage Learning. All Rights Reserved. May not be scanned, copied or duplicated, or posted to a publicly accessible website, in whole or in part.

CHAPTER 17

Written Communication

LEARNING OBJECTIVES

Studying and applying the material in this chapter will help you to:

- Explain why the ability to write clearly and correctly is an important skill for the health care professional.
- Describe effective techniques for planning and organizing written documents.
- Use correct spelling and grammar in all written communication.
- Explain how to write, format, and send effective business letters.
- List what should be included in meeting agendas and minutes.
- Describe techniques for creating effective written patient education materials.
- Discuss the proper handling of written documents to protect patient confidentiality.
- List ways to improve proofreading skills.

VOCABULARY REVIEW

Definitions

Write the definition of each of the following words or terms.

1. cross-training

____

____

____

2. etiquette

____

____

____

© 2017 Cengage Learning. All Rights Reserved. May not be scanned, copied or duplicated, or posted to a publicly accessible website, in whole or in part.

3. word processing

___

___

___

Matching

Match the following terms with their correct definitions.

____	1. agenda	A.	format in which first sentences of paragraphs are indented five spaces
____	2. modified block letter	B.	format in which all lines are even with the left margin
____	3. block letter	C.	greeting
____	4. justified	D.	text is lined up with a margin
____	5. semi-block letter	E.	list of what is to take place at a meeting
____	6. salutation	F.	format in which all lines are even with the left margin except the date, closing, and signature

Word Fill

Complete the following sentences by filling in the missing words.

contractions	independent clause	syllables	quotation
suffix	consonants	grammar	vowels

1. Most of the letters in the alphabet are ___________.
2. The words *it's* and *they've* are examples of ___________.
3. The set of rules that make up how a language is organized and structured is called ___________.
4. A/an ___________ contains a subject and a verb and can stand on its own.
5. Juan said, "I'm looking forward to graduating." This is an example of a/an ___________.
6. In the word *careful, ful* is the ___________.
7. The word *surgical* has three ___________.
8. The letters *a, e, i, o,* and *u* are ___________.

© 2017 Cengage Learning. All Rights Reserved. May not be scanned, copied or duplicated, or posted to a publicly accessible website, in whole or in part.

CHAPTER REVIEW

Identification

Place an "X" in front of the words that are spelled incorrectly.

_____ 1. abcess

_____ 2. address

_____ 3. association

_____ 4. cafeine

_____ 5. calender

_____ 6. deficiency

_____ 7. exercise

_____ 8. fatigue

_____ 9. Febuary

_____ 10. hieght

_____ 11. laboratory

_____ 12. lisence

_____ 13. occasionally

_____ 14. physicly

_____ 15. physician

_____ 16. pnuemonia

_____ 17. schedule

_____ 18. siezure

_____ 19. temperature

_____ 20. resuscitate

True/False

Indicate whether the following statements are true (T) or false (F).

_____ 1. Worrying about grammar and spelling is not really important when writing an email message.

_____ 2. A patient who receives a poorly written letter from a health care facility may question the competence of the health care professionals who work there.

_____ 3. It is not necessary to plan and organize short pieces of writing.

_____ 4. Errors in written documents can negatively affect patient care.

_____ 5. When brainstorming for writing ideas, don't waste time recording silly ideas.

_____ 6. Your own ideas can be a good source of information when you are gathering information to write a report.

_____ 7. It is recommended that writers always create a formal outline before beginning to write the first draft.

© 2017 Cengage Learning. All Rights Reserved. May not be scanned, copied or duplicated, or posted to a publicly accessible website, in whole or in part.

_____ 8. When working on a long report, it is recommended that you not try to write a perfect first draft.

_____ 9. Using a computerized spell-checker is a reliable way to check your spelling.

_____ 10. The difference between the block, modified block, and semi-block business letter formats is the level of importance of the content of the letters.

_____ 11. Inter-office memos should be written as carefully as letters sent to patients.

_____ 12. Minutes of meetings should include a list of who attended.

Multiple Choice

Circle the best answer for each of the following questions. There is only one correct answer to each question.

1. Which of the following is the correct rule for the placement of the letters *e* and *i* in a word?

   A. *e* before *i* except when *ei* sounds like *ay*
   B. *i* before *e* except when followed by another vowel
   C. *i* before *e* except after c

2. When adding a suffix to a word, which of the following applies?

   A. drop the final silent *e* if the suffix begins with a vowel
   B. drop the final silent *e* if the suffix begins with a consonant
   C. the letter *e* is never dropped

3. When is a final *y* changed to *ie?*

   A. whenever *s* is added to the word
   B. whenever *s* or *d* are added to the word
   C. whenever *s* or *d* are added and *y* is preceded by a consonant

4. The letter *k* is added to words ending in ___________ when adding suffixes that begin with *e, i,* or *y*.

   A. c
   B. s
   C. x

5. Which of the following plural forms is written correctly?

   A. potatos
   B. ratioes
   C. tomatoes

6. Which of the following acronyms is written correctly?

   A. cpr
   B. CPR
   C. Cpr

© 2017 Cengage Learning. All Rights Reserved. May not be scanned, copied or duplicated, or posted to a publicly accessible website, in whole or in part.

7. Which of the following sentences is punctuated correctly?
   A. When Juan graduated from his respiratory therapy program he found a good job at a local hospital.
   B. When Juan graduated from his respiratory therapy program, he found a good job at a local hospital.
   C. When Juan graduated from his respiratory therapy program; he found a good job at a local hospital.
8. Which of the following sentences is punctuated correctly?
   A. Sam wanted to lose weight, and get fit, so he joined a local gym.
   B. Sam wanted to lose weight and get fit, so he joined a local gym.
   C. Sam wanted to lose weight and get fit so he joined a local gym.
9. Which of the following sentences is punctuated correctly?
   A. The urgent care center that takes emergency cases like yours is on Elm Street.
   B. The urgent care center, that takes emergency cases like yours is on Elm Street.
   C. The urgent care center, that takes emergency cases like yours, is on Elm Street.
10. Which of the following sentences is punctuated correctly?
    A. The following foods are recommended for a heart healthy diet, fruits, vegetables, and fish.
    B. The following foods are recommended for a heart healthy diet; fruits, vegetables, and fish.
    C. The following foods are recommended for a heart healthy diet: fruits, vegetables, and fish.
11. Which of the following sentences is punctuated correctly?
    A. The assignment for today is to read the chapter titled "Plastic and Reconstructive Surgery."
    B. The assignment for today is to read the chapter titled "Plastic and Reconstructive Surgery".
    C. The assignment for today, is to read the chapter titled "Plastic and Reconstructive Surgery."
12. Which of the following sentences is punctuated correctly?
    A. Its going to be posted on the bulletin board.
    B. It's going to be posted on the bulletin board.
    C. Its' going to be posted on the bulletin board.

Short Answer

Read each question. Think about the information presented in the text, and then answer each question.

1. Why is writing correctly an important skill for the health care professional?

   ____

   ____

   ____

© 2017 Cengage Learning. All Rights Reserved. May not be scanned, copied or duplicated, or posted to a publicly accessible website, in whole or in part.

2. List four common purposes of a written document.

3. What are the three basic parts of a written document?

4. When would it be appropriate to use medical terminology in a letter?

5. Who might benefit most from using a mind map to organize their content for a writing assignment?

6. What is a possible consequence of misspelled words in a medical report?

7. List five types of letters that might be sent from a physician's office.

8. What are four reasons for taking minutes at meetings?

9. What is a good technique for proofreading that helps you concentrate on the appearance of words?

© 2017 Cengage Learning. All Rights Reserved. May not be scanned, copied or duplicated, or posted to a publicly accessible website, in whole or in part.

10. What are the eight points listed in the chapter's *Written Communication Checklist* that should serve as guidelines for all written materials?

____

____

____

Critical Thinking Scenarios

Read each scenario. Think about the information presented in the text, and then answer each question.

1. Cameron is studying to be a biomedical technician. He enjoys working with tools and troubleshooting problems, but can see no reason why he should worry about his writing skills.

   A. When might Cameron use writing skills in his career as a biomedical technician?

   ____

   ____

   ____

   B. What might be the consequences of his poor writing skills?

   ____

   ____

   ____

2. Maria is studying for her associate's degree and is currently taking an English class to fulfill a general education requirement. The current assignment is to write a ten-page research report on a health-related topic.

   A. What steps should Maria take as she prepares to write her report?

   ____

   ____

   ____

   B. After she has gathered information, into what three parts should she organize her content?

   ____

   ____

   ____

   C. What should she look for as she proofreads her final draft?

   ____

   ____

   ____

© 2017 Cengage Learning. All Rights Reserved. May not be scanned, copied or duplicated, or posted to a publicly accessible website, in whole or in part.

CHAPTER 18

Computers and Technology in Health Care

LEARNING OBJECTIVES

Studying and applying the material in this chapter will help you to:

- Explain why it is important for today's health care professional to be computer literate.
- Describe how computers and technology are applied in the following areas of health care:
  - Information management
  - Electronic health records
  - Creation of documents
  - Numerical calculations
  - Diagnostics
  - Treatment
  - Patient monitoring
  - Research
  - Education
  - Communication
- Explain the difference between computer hardware and software.
- Describe how to properly handle and maintain hardware components.
- Identify and describe the two major types of data storage.
- List six important guidelines for using computers effectively.
- Explain precautions that the health care professional can take to ensure computer security.
- List ways that the health care professional can acquire computer skills.

© 2017 Cengage Learning. All Rights Reserved. May not be scanned, copied or duplicated, or posted to a publicly accessible website, in whole or in part.

VOCABULARY REVIEW

Definitions

Write the definition of each of the following words or terms.

1. bioinformatics

2. computer literate

3. plagiarism

4. point-of-care charting

5. site license

6. cloud storage

© 2017 Cengage Learning. All Rights Reserved. May not be scanned, copied or duplicated, or posted to a publicly accessible website, in whole or in part.

Matching 1

Match the following terms with their correct definitions.

_____	1. CD-ROM	A.	focused light rays that can cut and remove tissue
_____	2. central processing unit	B.	workspace in the computer that stores data while the computer is turned on
_____	3. fiber optics	C.	component of the computer that manages and performs operations
_____	4. hard drive	D.	linked computers that communicate and share data
_____	5. hardware	E.	permanent data storage device
_____	6. lasers	F.	devices attached to computers
_____	7. networks	G.	optical disk that stores data
_____	8. peripherals	H.	physical components of a computer
_____	9. RAM	I.	technology in which data are transmitted via thin cables

Matching 2

Match the following terms with their correct definitions.

_____	1. download	A.	creating and sending messages from one computer to another
_____	2. electronic mail	B.	worldwide system of networked computers
_____	3. gateways	C.	groups of individuals who use the Internet to communicate and share information
_____	4. Internet	D.	software program that searches for and retrieves documents from the Internet
_____	5. key words	E.	lists of and links to Web pages
_____	6. search engine	F.	websites that serve mainly to provide links to other websites
_____	7. telemedicine	G.	to transfer files from the Internet onto one's computer
_____	8. virtual communities	H.	practice of medicine via phone lines
_____	9. computer virus	I.	term or phrase used to search for specific information on the Web
_____	10. Web directories	J.	software that contains instructions to perform destructive operations

© 2017 Cengage Learning. All Rights Reserved. May not be scanned, copied or duplicated, or posted to a publicly accessible website, in whole or in part.

Word Fill

Complete the following sentences by filling in the missing words.

artificial intelligence	electronic spreadsheets	software	record
application programs	database	files	fields
expert systems			

1. Word processing software and antivirus programs are examples of ________________.
2. Technology that enables computers to make decisions that we previously believed could be made only by humans is called ________________.
3. Organizing data in structured ways so they can be easily accessed can be done with ________________ software.
4. ________________ enable(s) users to perform numerical calculations.
5. Specialized collections of computerized data that assist physicians in diagnostics and treatments are called ________________.
6. ________________ are categories set up in a database to help organize information.
7. Groups of related computerized records are called ________________.
8. The term for describing a collection of related data is a/an ________________.
9. Without ________________, a computer is like a CD player without a D, unable to perform any operations.

CHAPTER REVIEW

True/False

Indicate whether the following statements are true (T) or false (F).

_____ 1. More than half of the hospitals in the United States have a comprehensive electronic records system in place.

_____ 2. Software is now available that converts spoken words to text.

_____ 3. Health care professionals who provide direct patient care, such as nurses, have very few tasks that require using a computer.

_____ 4. The federal government is encouraging the use of electronic medical records to increase efficiency and decrease the cost of health care.

_____ 5. Submitting Medicare claims electronically is voluntary.

_____ 6. Some physicians are concerned that electronic medical records are subject to errors and may compromise patient care.

_____ 7. Reports created from voice dictation software are nearly as accurate as reports transcribed from written documents.

_____ 8. Database software is helpful for exploring future scenarios, such as how many physical therapists to hire for a new rehabilitation hospital.

_____ 9. New tracking methods have reduced adverse reactions to prescription drugs to nearly zero.

_____ 10. It is illegal for employers to check activity on workplace computers, including emails, of their employees.

© 2017 Cengage Learning. All Rights Reserved. May not be scanned, copied or duplicated, or posted to a publicly accessible website, in whole or in part.

Matching 3

Match the following terms with the short descriptions.

_____	1. antivirus software	A.	allows the dispensing of drugs at off-site locations
_____	2. laptop	B.	provides means of communication between homebound individuals
_____	3. app	C.	automatically distributes e-mails on specific topics
_____	4. password	D.	consists of CPU and peripherals in one unit
_____	5. RAM	E.	enables computer to perform specialized tasks
_____	6. virtual community	F.	temporarily stores information in the computer
_____	7. site license	G.	gives permission to install software on more than one computer
_____	8. download	H.	prevents destructive instructions from invading your computer
_____	9. mailing list	I.	legislation that addresses the privacy of medical records
_____	10. telepharmacy	J.	when creating this, do not choose something obvious
_____	11. application program	K.	never do this with files if you don't know who sent them
_____	12. HIPAA	L.	computer program for use on mobile devices

Short Answer

Read each question. Think about the information presented in the text, and then answer each question.

1. What is the meaning of computer literacy and why is it important for health care professionals to be computer literate?

   ____

   ____

   ____

2. How is database technology applied in health care?

   ____

   ____

   ____

3. What are the uses and benefits of telemedicine?

   ____

   ____

   ____

© 2017 Cengage Learning. All Rights Reserved. May not be scanned, copied or duplicated, or posted to a publicly accessible website, in whole or in part.

4. What were the goals of the Human Genome Project?

5. List six recommendations for the care and maintenance of computer equipment.

6. What does MEDLINE, maintained by the National Library of Medicine, contain?

7. How have computers decreased the time needed for obtaining the Food and Drug Administration's approval of new pharmaceutical products?

8. How does virtual reality technology enable surgeons to perform better?

9. What are some examples of the use of remote diagnostics?

10. List six guidelines for evaluating the reliability of a website.

© 2017 Cengage Learning. All Rights Reserved. May not be scanned, copied or duplicated, or posted to a publicly accessible website, in whole or in part.

Completion

Use the words in the list to complete the following statements:

computed tomography	expert system	determine brain function	fiber optics
lasers	electronic chip	electrical impedance tomography	robotic surgery
image-guided	magnetic resonance imaging	sound waves	artificial intelligence

1. The diagnostic technique that takes X-rays from various angles and is used to evaluate soft tissue is called ________________.
2. A common use of this diagnostic tool in which a radioactive substance is injected into the patient is to ________________.
3. ________________ is an experimental diagnostic technique in which electrodes are attached to the patient's skin.
4. The activity of hydrogen atoms in tissues is the basis for ________________.
5. ATHENA is an example of a/an ________________.
6. Ultrasonography uses ________________ in place of X-rays to create images of organs and abnormalities.
7. Some dentists use computer technology by placing a/an ________________ in the patient's mouth to send an image to a computer.
8. Hair-thin cables transmit data in a technology called ________________.
9. The sophisticated technology that helps health care professionals make decisions is ________________.
10. Cameras that provide high-resolution, three-dimensional images are used to perform ________________.
11. Highly focused light rays, called ________________, are now used to make precise cuts in tissue.
12. ________________ surgery is very accurate because it is based on a three-dimensional mapping system and technology that reports the exact location of surgical instruments.

Critical Thinking Scenarios

Read each scenario. Think about the information presented in the text, and then answer each question.

1. Ed had an appointment with Dr. Cardoza today about pain he's been experiencing in his abdomen. Dr. Cardoza noted a lump in Ed's abdomen and is arranging for him to have an MRI. On the way out of the office, Ed expressed concerns about the procedure to Addison, Dr. Cardoza's medical assistant.

   A. Why might Dr. Cardoza have recommended an MRI rather than another type of imaging?

   ____

   ____

   ____

© 2017 Cengage Learning. All Rights Reserved. May not be scanned, copied or duplicated, or posted to a publicly accessible website, in whole or in part.

B. What happens during the procedure?

C. How can Addison help Ed feel more comfortable about having an MRI?

2. Jeb is a newly graduated surgical technologist. He wants to learn more about the developing field of robotics and how they are used in surgery.

   A. Where might he locate the most current information?

   B. What key words might be useful for finding information on the Internet?

   C. What types of websites generally have the most reliable information?

© 2017 Cengage Learning. All Rights Reserved. May not be scanned, copied or duplicated, or posted to a publicly accessible website, in whole or in part.

CHAPTER 19

Documentation and Medical Records

LEARNING OBJECTIVES

Studying and applying the material in this chapter will help you to:

- State the primary responsibility of the health care professional regarding the regulations of Health Insurance Portability and Accountability Act of 1996.
- List and explain the purposes of medical documentation.
- List the characteristics of good medical documentation.
- Explain the proper method for correcting errors on medical records.
- List the various sources of information that may be found in a medical record.
- Describe three different formats used for progress notes.
- Discuss the advantages and disadvantages of each progress note format.
- Discuss advantages of an electronic health record (EHR) coordinated system.
- Describe what information would be included in a personal health record (PHR).

© 2017 Cengage Learning. All Rights Reserved. May not be scanned, copied or duplicated, or posted to a publicly accessible website, in whole or in part.

VOCABULARY REVIEW

Matching 1

Match the following terms with their correct definitions.

	Term		Definition
_____	1. assessment	A.	recording observations and information about patients
_____	2. charting	B.	a format for charting that uses a problem-oriented approach
_____	3. chief complaint	C.	gathering information; a step in charting that is the health care professional's impression of what is wrong with the patient, based on the signs and symptoms
_____	4. medical documentation	D.	written chronological statements about a patient's care
_____	5. medical history	E.	the patient's statement of the main reason he or she is seeking medical care
_____	6. medical record	F.	a step in SOAP charting that documents the procedures, treatments, and patient instructions that make up the patient's care
_____	7. plan	G.	notes and documents that health care professionals add to the medical record
_____	8. progress notes	H.	the collection of all documents that are filed together and form a complete chronological health history of a particular patient
_____	9. SOAP	I.	data collected on a patient that includes personal, familial, and social information

CHAPTER REVIEW

True/False

Indicate whether the following statements are true (T) or false (F).

_____ 1. An example of medical documentation would be patient statistics and information about care.

_____ 2. Charting is the process of administering care.

_____ 3. A medical record refers to a section of personal notes made by the physician only.

_____ 4. Many health care professionals are responsible for some aspect of charting.

_____ 5. Patient comments should not be included in a medical record; only observations made by health care professional should be included.

_____ 6. Complete and accurate medical documentation is critical in providing consistent patient care.

© 2017 Cengage Learning. All Rights Reserved. May not be scanned, copied or duplicated, or posted to a publicly accessible website, in whole or in part.

_____ 7. Information included in the medical record is a significant source of data on which other health care professionals can base their approach to the patient.

_____ 8. The medical record is not a legal document and as such cannot be used in a court of law.

_____ 9. The security of records is the responsibility of each health care professional.

_____ 10. The progress notes make up the written record of every aspect of a patient's relationship with the health care professional.

_____ 11. Computers are being increasingly used in the health care field.

_____ 12. Electronic health records (EHR) offer less options for information than core charting.

_____ 13. The computerized systems can also include many informational and safety tools.

_____ 14. Personal health records (PHRs) are becoming increasingly important due to the mobility of individuals and frequent changes in health care providers.

_____ 15. HIPAA is a private accreditation agency that makes site visits to facilities.

Matching 2

Match the following terms with their correct definitions.

	Term		Definition
_____	1. source-oriented record format	A.	forms for specialty needs
_____	2. continuous chronological record format	B.	record is divided into different sections by specialty
_____	3. familial history	C.	when the primary physician asks another physician to see the patient
_____	4. social history	D.	if and how much a patient smokes, drinks alcohol, or takes illegal drugs
_____	5. personal history	E.	when the physician dictates findings and then they are typed from the taped message
_____	6. consultation	F.	all documentation organized by date entered
_____	7. transcription services	G.	patient's past medical problems and surgeries, allergies, and so on
_____	8. flow sheets	H.	includes all medications administered by health care professionals at the facility
_____	9. medication record	I.	medical problems of relatives
_____	10. progress notes	J.	written chronological statements about a patient's care

© 2017 Cengage Learning. All Rights Reserved. May not be scanned, copied or duplicated, or posted to a publicly accessible website, in whole or in part.

Short Answer

Read each question. Think about the information presented in the text, and then answer each question.

1. List the characteristics of good medical documentation.

2. What does it mean when it is stated that charting needs to be clearly and objectively expressed?

3. Why is it important that the health care professional uses correct spelling, terminology, punctuation, and grammar when charting?

4. When should charting be completed? Why?

5. When is the appropriate time to chart a medication or procedure?

6. What are the proper steps to take when correcting a written documentation?

7. Give an example of when a flow sheet may be used.

8. What are graphic forms used for?

© 2017 Cengage Learning. All Rights Reserved. May not be scanned, copied or duplicated, or posted to a publicly accessible website, in whole or in part.

9. What are diagnostic tests?

____

____

____

10. What is included in physician's orders?

____

____

____

Completion

Use the words in the list to complete the following statements:

"thinning the chart"	done	subjective	JCAHO
medical history	objective	problem-oriented	narrative
evaluation	charting by exception (CBE)		

1. Only through written documentation can tests, procedures, and treatment be proven to have occurred. In the world of health care, "If it isn't documented, it isn't _______________."
2. _______________ is an accreditation organization for health care facilities.
3. A/An _______________ includes the personal, familial, and social history of a patient.
4. _______________ is done when the chart becomes too thick and another file on the patient is started.
5. _______________ medical records are organized around the patient's health problems.
6. _______________ information is that which is sensed and reported by the patient.
7. _______________ information includes observations of health care professionals.
8. A/An _______________ is done to determine what the results were and if the treatment was effective.
9. _______________ charting includes detailed written notes on all aspects of care.
10. _______________ is an abbreviated chart format where only abnormal findings are noted.

© 2017 Cengage Learning. All Rights Reserved. May not be scanned, copied or duplicated, or posted to a publicly accessible website, in whole or in part.

Critical Thinking Scenarios

Read each scenario. Think about the information presented in the text, and then answer each question.

1. Mrs. Gonzales comes into the clinic and says her husband asked her to stop by to get information as to when his next appointment is scheduled.

   A. Can this information be given to Mrs. Gonzales?

   ____

   ____

   ____

   B. Why or why not?

   ____

   ____

   ____

   C. What are the possible consequences if correct protocol is not followed?

   ____

   ____

   ____

2. Ms. Sally Jessups has read an article about creating a personal health record. She wonders if this is something she should put together.

   A. What reasons might she want to consider in her decision?

   ____

   ____

   ____

   B. What type of information should this record include?

   ____

   ____

   ____

   C. What are the advantages of having a personal health record?

   ____

   ____

   ____

© 2017 Cengage Learning. All Rights Reserved. May not be scanned, copied or duplicated, or posted to a publicly accessible website, in whole or in part.

UNIT 7
Health Care Skills

© 2017 Cengage Learning. All Rights Reserved. May not be scanned, copied or duplicated, or posted to a publicly accessible website, in whole or in part.

CHAPTER 20

Physical Assessment

LEARNING OBJECTIVES

Studying and applying the material in this chapter will help you to:

- State the purpose of a history and physical (H&P) and indicate what data the physician will obtain.
- Discuss variances from the norm for each of the body systems.
- Discuss the value of using a pain scale.
- Define what actions are included in the activities of daily living (ADLs).
- Correctly take the vital signs (temperature, pulse, respirations, and blood pressure).
- Describe how the presence of an apical-radial deficit is determined and what it means.
- Measure the height and weight of a patient.

VOCABULARY REVIEW

Matching 1

Match the following terms with their correct definitions.

	Term	Definition
_____	1. afebrile	A. a respiratory rate that is below the normal range
_____	2. apnea	B. breathing that is within the normal range, is unlabored, and has an even rhythm
_____	3. bradycardia	C. blood pressure below the normal range
_____	4. bradypnea	D. absence of respirations
_____	5. Cheyne-Stokes	E. a temperature that is within the normal range
_____	6. dyspnea	F. blood pressure above the normal range
_____	7. eupnea	G. the part of the respiratory cycle when air enters the lungs
_____	8. exhalation	H. the part of the respiratory cycle when air is removed from the lungs
_____	9. hypertension	I. a heart rate that is below the normal rate
_____	10. hypotension	J. a breathing pattern that has a period of apnea followed by a gradually increasing depth and frequency of respirations
_____	11. inhalation	K. labored breathing or difficulty with breathing

© 2017 Cengage Learning. All Rights Reserved. May not be scanned, copied or duplicated, or posted to a publicly accessible website, in whole or in part.

Matching 2

Match the following definitions with their correct terms.

	Definition		Term
_____	1. the process of taking air into and removing air from the lungs	A.	febrile
_____	2. a temperature that is elevated above the normal range	B.	orthopnea
_____	3. an instrument that amplifies sounds so they can be heard from within the body	C.	orthostatic (postural) hypotension
_____	4. when a patient has difficulty breathing unless in a sitting or standing position	D.	pulse deficit
_____	5. a heart rate that is above the normal range	E.	pulse points
_____	6. the difference between a pulse point and an apical rate that are taken simultaneously	F.	respiration
_____	7. an instrument that records the blood pressure	G.	stethoscope
_____	8. a respiratory rate that is above the normal range	H.	sphygmomanometer
_____	9. the rapid lowering of the blood pressure as a result of changing positions	I.	tachycardia
_____	10. measuring the blood pressure, temperature, pulse, and respiration to give some indication of how the body is functioning	J.	tachypnea
_____	11. specific sites on the body where arterial pulsations can be felt	K.	vital signs

© 2017 Cengage Learning. All Rights Reserved. May not be scanned, copied or duplicated, or posted to a publicly accessible website, in whole or in part.

CHAPTER REVIEW

Identification

Place an "X" in front of the items of information that are included in the patient's H&P.

_____ 1. demographic date

_____ 2. date

_____ 3. chief complaint

_____ 4. history of present illness

_____ 5. current health status

_____ 6. criminal record

_____ 7. source of referral

_____ 8. family history of illness

_____ 9. review of all systems

_____ 10. psychosocial history

True/False Rewrite

Please rewrite the bold part of the sentence to make the statement true.

1. The **admission office personnel** takes a history and performs a physical on patients when they are seen for the first time or when they are admitted to the hospital.

____

____

____

2. Demographic data include **general state of the patient's health**.

____

____

____

3. A source of referral is a **list of all prior hospitalizations**.

____

____

____

4. A chief complaint is the primary problem from the **physician's view** as to why the patient is seeking medical care.

____

____

____

© 2017 Cengage Learning. All Rights Reserved. May not be scanned, copied or duplicated, or posted to a publicly accessible website, in whole or in part.

5. The observational skills needed are based on a thorough understanding of **etiology and pathophysiology**.

6. **Percussion** refers to the use of the senses of vision, hearing, and smell for observation of patient condition.

7. A patient's gait refers to **the status of his or her skin**.

8. Assessing capillary refill is when the health care professional **inspects the neck veins for distention**.

9. Menarche means **menopause**.

10. An axillary temperature will be a **higher** than an oral temperature.

Multiple Choice

Circle the best answer for each of the following questions. There is only one correct answer to each question.

1. Which of the following means a temperature is elevated above the normal range?

   A. febrile
   B. afebrile
   C. intermittent fever

© 2017 Cengage Learning. All Rights Reserved. May not be scanned, copied or duplicated, or posted to a publicly accessible website, in whole or in part.

2. What creates the pulsing sensation felt by health care professionals at certain points in the body?

   A. the coronary arteries contracting
   B. the heart valves opening
   C. the heart contracting

3. What is the name of the type of pulse being taken when a stethoscope is used to listen to the heart beat?

   A. carotid
   B. apical
   C. radial

4. What creates the sound of "lub-dub" heard when a stethoscope is placed over the heart?

   A. heart contracting
   B. valves closing
   C. flow of blood

5. What is the normal range for the pulse of an adult?

   A. 60–80 beats per minute
   B. 60–90 beats per minute
   C. 80–100 beats per minute

6. If the apical pulse if 90 and the radial pulse is 50, what is the pulse deficit?

   A. 40
   B. 50
   C. 90

7. What is the normal respiratory range for an adult?

   A. 22–34 breaths per minute
   B. 18–24 breaths per minute
   C. 16–20 breaths per minute

8. Which number is the diastolic if the blood pressure is 134/76 and the pulse is 84?

   A. 134
   B. 76
   C. 84

9. What is white coat syndrome?

   A. when patients want to make their own diagnoses
   B. increased blood pressure during office visits
   C. a fear of white

10. Which of the following would be a reason not to use an arm for a blood pressure reading?

   A. Patient had mastectomy on that side
   B. Patient recently had abdominal surgery
   C. Patient recently had blood drawn in that arm

© 2017 Cengage Learning. All Rights Reserved. May not be scanned, copied or duplicated, or posted to a publicly accessible website, in whole or in part.

Short Answer

Read each question. Think about the information presented in the text, and then answer each question.

1. What is meant by doing a general survey and why is it done?

2. What should be included in a psychosocial evaluation?

3. What are the skills frequently used during the physical evaluation of the patient?

4. Explain the two primary methods used to evaluate pain.

5. What are ADLs?

6. When taking a pulse, what three observations are made?

7. When taking a respiratory rate, what three observations are made?

8. How do vital signs vary over the life span?

© 2017 Cengage Learning. All Rights Reserved. May not be scanned, copied or duplicated, or posted to a publicly accessible website, in whole or in part.

9. List the four methods commonly used to record a patient's weight.

____

____

____

10. If you need a patient's height but he or she cannot stand, what do you do?

____

____

____

Ordering 1

Place the following duties in the order in which they should be performed when doing a head-to-toe assessment on an adult. Put a numeral 1 before the first duty, a 2 before the next, and so on.

_____ 1. chest (respiratory and cardiac symptoms)

_____ 2. orientation

_____ 3. neck

_____ 4. head

_____ 5. abdomen

_____ 6. upper extremities

_____ 7. lower extremities

Ordering 2

Place the following duties in the order in which they should be performed when taking a manual blood pressure. Put a numeral 1 before the first duty, a 2 before the next, and so on.

_____ 1. Add 30 to the reading obtained in the prior step

_____ 2. Deflate cuff until can no longer hear any sounds

_____ 3. Locate brachial artery

_____ 4. Inflate cuff until cannot feel radial artery

_____ 5. Deflate cuff until hear first sound

_____ 6. Inflate cuff to predetermined amount

_____ 7. Place stethoscope over brachial artery

_____ 8. Record readings

_____ 9. Deflate cuff and remove from arm

_____ 10. Deflate cuff and wait 30 sec

© 2017 Cengage Learning. All Rights Reserved. May not be scanned, copied or duplicated, or posted to a publicly accessible website, in whole or in part.

Labeling

Assign the labels in the list to the appropriate places on the figure where they can be felt on the body.

Figure 20–1 Pulse Points

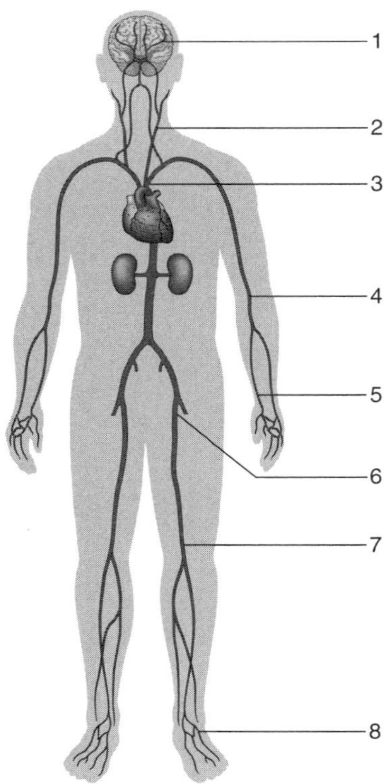

_____ popliteal artery
_____ temporal artery
_____ dorsalis pedis artery
_____ femoral artery
_____ brachial artery
_____ apex (apical pulse)
_____ carotid artery
_____ radial artery

Critical Thinking Scenarios

Read each scenario. Think about the information presented in the text, and then answer each question.

1. During a physical examination of a patient the physician notes a decreased ROM of the patient's upper extremities.

   A. What is the system that is most likely being referred to in this finding?

   ____

   ____

   ____

   B. What does ROM stand for?

   ____

   ____

   ____

© 2017 Cengage Learning. All Rights Reserved. May not be scanned, copied or duplicated, or posted to a publicly accessible website, in whole or in part.

C. How is it assessed?

2. Mr. Andrews is complaining about shortness of breath. He says he feels like he just cannot get enough oxygen. He is a dark-skinned patient and so it is difficult to determine if he is cyanotic or not.

   A. What does cyanotic mean?

   B. How do you assess for cyanosis in a Caucasian?

   C. How do you assess for cyanosis in a dark-skinned patient?

   D. What system is compromised in this scenario?

Health Care Procedures

Complete the procedures for this chapter at the end of the workbook.

© 2017 Cengage Learning. All Rights Reserved. May not be scanned, copied or duplicated, or posted to a publicly accessible website, in whole or in part.

CHAPTER 21

Emergency Procedures

LEARNING OBJECTIVES

Studying and applying the material in this chapter will help you to:

- Explain when first aid should be administered.
- Discuss how the Good Samaritan Act protects the rescuer.
- State the golden rule of first aid.
- Understand the seven steps to follow that will protect both the victim and rescuer when an emergency occurs.
- Identify when CPR should be performed.
- Identify illnesses and injuries that may require first aid, including their signs and symptoms and treatment.
- Demonstrate the proper application of slings and spiral, figure-eight, and finger wraps.

© 2017 Cengage Learning. All Rights Reserved. May not be scanned, copied or duplicated, or posted to a publicly accessible website, in whole or in part.

VOCABULARY REVIEW

Matching

Match the following terms with their correct definitions.

_____	1. anaphylactic shock	A.	when blood drains to the outside of the body through a break in the skin
_____	2. cardiopulmonary resuscitation (CPR)	B.	a primary principle when assisting others, meaning to "do no further harm"
_____	3. closed fracture	C.	condition in which the body temperature is above the normal range
_____	4. external bleeding	D.	manually providing respiratory and cardiac support for a patient who is not breathing and whose heart has stopped beating
_____	5. first aid	E.	a life-threatening severe allergic reaction resulting in swelling of the respiratory system that restricts breathing
_____	6. frostbite	F.	severe, heavy bleeding
_____	7. golden rule	G.	condition in which the body temperature is below the normal range
_____	8. Good Samaritan Act	H.	a law to protect individuals from liability when they stop to assist someone who has been hurt or is ill
_____	9. hemorrhage	I.	when a bone is broken but does not protrude through the skin
_____	10. hyperthermia	J.	emergency care provided to an accident victim or to someone who has become suddenly ill
_____	11. hypothermia	K.	condition in which the skin begins to freeze

Word Fill

Complete the following sentences by filling in the missing words.

internal bleeding	joint dislocation	Medic Alert	open fracture
rescue breathing	rescuer	sprains	strains
sucking wound	victim	wound	

1. A/An __________________ is a person giving care during an emergency.
2. __________________ is when blood loss occurs inside the body.
3. __________________ are torn ligament fibers that result in a loosening of the joint.
4. __________________ is when a joint becomes disconnected from its socket.
5. A/An __________________ is a puncture into the respiratory system resulting in loss of air as the patient breathes.
6. A/An __________________ is when a broken bone protrudes through the skin.

© 2017 Cengage Learning. All Rights Reserved. May not be scanned, copied or duplicated, or posted to a publicly accessible website, in whole or in part.

7. ________________ are the result of sudden tearing of muscle fibers during exertion; also referred to as a pulled muscle.
8. A/An ________________ is a person requiring care during an emergency.
9. ________________ is an organization that provides bracelets or pendants for patients to wear that contain information or warnings about specific medical problems.
10. A/An ________________ is damage to the soft tissue of the body as a result of violence or trauma.
11. ________________ is a technique in which the rescuer breathes for the victim.

CHAPTER REVIEW

True/False

Indicate whether the following statements are true (T) or false (F).

_____ 1. First aid refers to providing emergency care to an accident victim or to someone who has suddenly become ill.

_____ 2. The American Red Cross (ARC) recommends that all health care professionals take a first aid and safety course, but it is not necessary for the general public.

_____ 3. The Good Samaritan Act requires someone to assist if they come across a victim in need of assistance.

_____ 4. You can attempt procedures you do not have the skills to perform if you feel the victim may benefit from trying.

_____ 5. Before approaching the victim, assess the situation to determine if it is safe to approach.

_____ 6. If there are hazards that would put the Good Samaritan at risk, the appropriate course of action is to not approach, but to call for help immediately.

_____ 7. Even in an emergency situation, a person has the right to refuse care.

_____ 8. Do not assume what might have occurred. If the victim is conscious, ask for information.

_____ 9. Standard precautions do not apply to emergency situations.

_____ 10. CPR, if needed, is always the first priority in any situation where first aid emergency care is given.

Multiple Choice

Circle the best answer for each of the following questions. There is only one correct answer to each question.

1. When is CPR administered?

   A. When someone is breathing but has no pulse
   B. When someone is not breathing but has a pulse
   C. When someone is not breathing and does not have a pulse

© 2017 Cengage Learning. All Rights Reserved. May not be scanned, copied or duplicated, or posted to a publicly accessible website, in whole or in part.

2. When is it appropriate to move an accident victim?
   A. If he or she gives you permission
   B. If the victim's life is in immediate danger if not moved
   C. If you can give better first aid in another location
3. Obtaining CPR training results in what type of recognition?
   A. A certificate
   B. A license
   C. An award
4. Which of the following is true about allergic reactions?
   A. They are mild and can easily be treated with an antihistamine
   B. They are life threatening and EMS should be called at the first sign of a reaction
   C. They can range from mild to life threatening
5. If a victim was stung and the stinger is visible, what is the best action to follow?
   A. Remove it by squeezing it from both sides
   B. Leave it in place
   C. Remove it by using a fingernail or credit card to scrape across it
6. What should the rescuer do if internal bleeding is suspected?
   A. Apply ice
   B. Call EMS
   C. Monitor to see if it is serious
7. What should the rescuer do if there is external bleeding?
   A. Apply pressure
   B. Check wound frequently to see if it has subsided
   C. Apply a tourniquet
8. What should the rescuer do when treating large wounds?
   A. Remove embedded objects and clean as much as possible
   B. Apply a tourniquet
   C. Remove any obvious loose debris from the wound
9. What is the characteristic of a sucking wound?
   A. Bubbling from the wound
   B. Spurting of blood from the wound
   C. Extreme pain
10. What should the rescuer do with an amputated part?
    A. It is not important as reattachment is not likely
    B. Pack it in ice
    C. Keep it with the victim
11. What is the purpose of a sling?
    A. Apply pressure to a wound
    B. Support injured leg, foot, or knee
    C. Support injured shoulder, collarbone, or arm

© 2017 Cengage Learning. All Rights Reserved. May not be scanned, copied or duplicated, or posted to a publicly accessible website, in whole or in part.

12. Where should the knot of a sling be tied?
    A. Over a bone
    B. Over soft tissue
    C. It doesn't matter
13. What is the purpose of a spiral wrap?
    A. Enhance circulation and decrease swelling
    B. Used instead of a tourniquet
    C. To restrict excessive bleeding
14. Where should you start a figure-eight wrap when applying it for an ankle injury?
    A. At the knee
    B. At the instep
    C. Midthigh
15. If the finger is broken, what should you do before applying the bandage to the finger?
    A. Apply a sling
    B. Apply a figure-eight wrap
    C. Apply a splint

Short Answer

Read each question. Think about the information presented in the text, and then answer each question.

1. What is the difference between a first-, second-, and third-degree burn?

____

____

____

2. Define drug abuse.

____

____

____

3. What should the rescuer do for a drug overdose?

____

____

____

4. What are the most common routes of poisonings?

____

____

____

© 2017 Cengage Learning. All Rights Reserved. May not be scanned, copied or duplicated, or posted to a publicly accessible website, in whole or in part.

5. What are the most common sites for frostbite?

___

___

___

6. How should the rescuer treat a victim with heat stroke?

___

___

___

7. What is the main goal in treating hyperventilation?

___

___

___

8. What is another name for chest pain? What causes it?

___

___

___

9. If the victim is diabetic and it is unclear whether she is hyperglycemic or hypoglycemic, what treatment should be administered? Why?

___

___

___

10. What are the three common types of seizures?

___

___

___

Completion

Use the words in the list to complete the following statements:

Medic Alert	golden rule	eye injury	tourniquet
depth	muscle strain	rescuer; victim	Heimlich maneuver
venous; arterial	calm		

1. The ________________ in providing first aid is to "do no further harm."
2. The person giving care is called a ________________ and the person requiring care is called the ________________.
3. A form of identification called ________________ may specify if the victim is diabetic, epileptic, or has specific heart problems or allergies.
4. A ________________, reassuring manner in treating a victim will decrease the stress of the situation for the victim.

© 2017 Cengage Learning. All Rights Reserved. May not be scanned, copied or duplicated, or posted to a publicly accessible website, in whole or in part.

5. If a victim has an obstructed airway, perform the ________________.
6. Do not ever apply a ________________ to an extremity.
7. Blood that flows evenly from an injury is ________________ bleeding. Blood that is a brighter red and comes out in spurts with each heartbeat is ________________ bleeding.
8. A pulled muscle is also called a ________________.
9. Any ________________ should always be taken very seriously because it can involve the loss of vision.
10. The severity of the burn is determined by the size, ________________, and location of the burn.

Critical Thinking Scenarios

Read each scenario. Think about the information presented in the text, and then answer each question.

1. Mr. Worthington has been in a car accident and is exhibiting signs of shock.
   A. What are the signs of shock?

   ____

   ____

   ____

   B. What causes shock?

   ____

   ____

   ____

   C. What can the rescuer do to assist the victim?

   ____

   ____

   ____

2. Mrs. Johnston falls to the floor at the mall due to sudden weakness on the left side of the body. The rescuer does an assessment and determines it is most likely a stroke.
   A. What causes a stroke?

   ____

   ____

   ____

   B. What is a TIA?

   ____

   ____

   ____

© 2017 Cengage Learning. All Rights Reserved. May not be scanned, copied or duplicated, or posted to a publicly accessible website, in whole or in part.

C. What should the rescuer do to assist the victim?

____

____

____

Health Care Procedures

Complete the procedures for this chapter at the end of the workbook.

© 2017 Cengage Learning. All Rights Reserved. May not be scanned, copied or duplicated, or posted to a publicly accessible website, in whole or in part.

UNIT 8
Business of Caring

© 2017 Cengage Learning. All Rights Reserved. May not be scanned, copied or duplicated, or posted to a publicly accessible website, in whole or in part.

CHAPTER 22

Controlling Health Care Costs

LEARNING OBJECTIVES

Studying and applying the material in this chapter will help you to:

- Identify factors that are causing an increase in health care costs.
- Identify the three types of funding for health care institutions.
- Compare and contrast the three types of payment methods.
- Describe how methods for paying medical costs have changed over the years.
- Contrast fee-for-service and managed care reimbursement methods.
- Explain the purpose of managed care systems and describe the methods used to control costs.
- Define Medicare, Medicaid, and diagnostic-related groups (DRGs).
- Identify the four major areas of expenditures incurred by a health care delivery system.
- Define accounts receivable, accounts payable, and the cost of money.
- Explain ways that the health care worker can help control facility costs.

VOCABULARY REVIEW

Definitions

Write the definition of each of the following words or terms.

1. accounts payable

____

____

____

2. accounts receivable

____

____

____

© 2017 Cengage Learning. All Rights Reserved. May not be scanned, copied or duplicated, or posted to a publicly accessible website, in whole or in part.

3. capitation

4. coinsurance

5. copay

6. cost of money

7. deductible

8. diagnostic-related group (DRG)

9. expenditures

10. fee-for-service

11. financing

© 2017 Cengage Learning. All Rights Reserved. May not be scanned, copied or duplicated, or posted to a publicly accessible website, in whole or in part.

Matching 1

Match the following terms with their correct definitions.

____	1. gatekeeper	A.	promotion of cost-effective health care through the management and control of its delivery
____	2. managed care	B.	federally funded insurance program for individuals aged 65 and older and others, such as the disabled, who qualify for Social Security
____	3. Medicaid	C.	a health care provider, often a physician, who serves as the patient's first contact when entering the health care system; also known as gatekeeper
____	4. Medicare	D.	approval from an insurance company prior to certain health care services, for the purposes of determining medical necessity and cost effectiveness
____	5. negotiated fees	E.	to pay back
____	6. preauthorization	F.	a health care provider, often a physician, who serves as the patient's first contact when entering the health care system; also known as primary care provider
____	7. premium	G.	federally funded but state-administered insurance plan for individuals who qualify due to low income
____	8. prepaid plans	H.	an agreed-upon amount paid to an insurance company for the benefit of having the company pay for a specified amount of future health care costs
____	9. primary care provider (PCP)	I.	amount negotiated between insurance companies and health care groups for the cost of services; depending on the plan, the patient either pays the difference in actual cost of service or the health care group accepts the predetermined amount as payment in full
____	10. profit	J.	a contracted type of insurance plan in which health care providers are paid a specific amount to provide certain health benefits
____	11. reimburse	K.	amount of money remaining after all costs of operating a business have been paid

© 2017 Cengage Learning. All Rights Reserved. May not be scanned, copied or duplicated, or posted to a publicly accessible website, in whole or in part.

CHAPTER REVIEW

Identification 1

Place an "X" in front of programs or regulations that are operated or initiated by the government.

_____ 1. Medicare

_____ 2. Medicaid

_____ 3. health maintenance organization (HMO)

_____ 4. exclusive provider organization (EPO)

_____ 5. preferred provider organization (PPO)

_____ 6. point-of-service plan (POS)

_____ 7. Medicare Prescription Drug, Improvement and Modernization Act (MMA) of 2003

_____ 8. diagnostic-related groups (DRGs)

Identification 2

Place an "X" in front of services that may apply to Part B of Medicare.

_____ 1. hospital stay

_____ 2. skilled facility following a hospital stay

_____ 3. outpatient medical supplies

_____ 4. inpatient diagnostic tests

_____ 5. hospice care

_____ 6. outpatient physical and occupational therapy

_____ 7. home health

_____ 8. outpatient prescription drugs

_____ 9. HMO or PPO organizations

_____ 10. physician's fee for office visit

True/False

Indicate whether the following statements are true (T) or false (F).

_____ 1. A major concern in the United States today is how to effectively control dramatically rising health care costs.

_____ 2. Health care costs are evenly distributed among all patients.

_____ 3. Chronic conditions are seen only in the aged.

_____ 4. More money is spent per person on health care in the United States than in any other country.

_____ 5. The youth of this nation are showing an alarming increase in obesity, poor diet, and lack of physical fitness.

© 2017 Cengage Learning. All Rights Reserved. May not be scanned, copied or duplicated, or posted to a publicly accessible website, in whole or in part.

_____ 6. Prepaid plans are based on the idea that providers can be motivated to be more efficient.

_____ 7. Insurance coverage is based on the concept that those who need the service will pay more.

_____ 8. Medicare is free and covers all medical expenses.

_____ 9. Medicare has a monthly premium along with deductibles and coinsurance amounts.

_____ 10. Medicaid is a cost-assistance program to help pay the medical costs for those who qualify due to low income.

Matching 2

Match the following terms with their correct definitions.

	Term		Definition
_____	1. HMO (health maintenance organization)	A.	greater flexibility than an HMO to create a benefits package specific to a company's needs
_____	2. EPO (exclusive provider organization)	B.	a group of hospitals and physicians who contract on a fee-for-service basis
_____	3. PPO (preferred provider organization)	C.	administered by the Centers for Medicare and Medicaid Services (CMS)
_____	4. POS (point-of-service plan)	D.	members can choose to receive a service from participating or nonparticipating providers
_____	5. another name for gatekeepers	E.	prepaid medical group practice plan that provides a predetermined medical care benefit package
_____	6. Medicare	F.	primary care providers (PCPs)
_____	7. Medigap	G.	often the largest cost incurred by a facility
_____	8. generic	H.	supplemental insurance policy for costs not included under Medicare
_____	9. accounts receivable	I.	these drugs are less expensive than brand names
_____	10. personnel	J.	a sound business practice is to keep this as low as possible

Short Answer

Read each question. Think about the information presented in the text, and then answer each question.

1. Why did the fee-for-service plan go out of favor?

____

____

____

© 2017 Cengage Learning. All Rights Reserved. May not be scanned, copied or duplicated, or posted to a publicly accessible website, in whole or in part.

2. List the three type of health care institutions with a brief description of each.

3. What is preauthorization? Why is it important for the health care professional to know when it is required?

4. What is the purpose of Medicare? What are Parts A, B, C, and D?

5. Explain how DRGs came about and how they work.

6. Health care facilities' expenditures occur in what four major areas?

7. List four ways that the health care professional can contribute to the efficient and cost-effective functioning of the facility.

8. What is the most likely cause when employees have difficulty performing efficiently?

9. How can the use of a problem-solving process help the employee improve efficiency?

© 2017 Cengage Learning. All Rights Reserved. May not be scanned, copied or duplicated, or posted to a publicly accessible website, in whole or in part.

10. What four questions can employees ask themselves in seeking to help reduce unnecessary costs?

    ____

    ____

    ____

11. List the three health care payment methods with a brief description of each.

    ____

    ____

    ____

Completion

Use the words in the list to complete the following statements.

physician; insurance company	prepaid	expenditures	premium
managed care	primary care providers (PCPs)	copay	financing resources
		capitation	profit

1. Paying an insurance company an agreed-upon amount for coverage is called a __________.
2. A fee-for-service plan is when the __________ determines what actions to take and the __________ pays for the services.
3. __________ plans contain specific built-in cost controls.
4. A __________ is the amount of money remaining after all costs of operating a business have been paid.
5. In __________ plans, health care providers are paid before rather than after services are performed.
6. When the provider is paid the same regardless of the type or number of services provided, the method of payment is called __________.
7. A __________ is paying a set amount for each visit or service.
8. One method that has been devised to reduce the overuse of services by patients is the use of __________.
9. __________ refer to any money that is spent in the process of doing business.
10. __________ for a health care facility come primarily from a variety of health insurance companies.

© 2017 Cengage Learning. All Rights Reserved. May not be scanned, copied or duplicated, or posted to a publicly accessible website, in whole or in part.

Critical Thinking Scenarios

Read each scenario. Think about the information presented in the text, and then answer each question.

1. Maria Torres just started working in a new health care facility. She notes that her coworkers take excessive breaks and is concerned about the impact it has on patient care.

   A. What impact does her coworkers' behavior have on Maria?

   ____

   ____

   ____

   B. What impact does her coworkers' behavior have on patient care?

   ____

   ____

   ____

   C. What impact does it have on the facility's ability to function?

   ____

   ____

   ____

2. Mr. Gerald Beuller is trying to decide what insurance policy he should choose. He finds it very confusing and angrily states "between the deductibles, copays, and coinsurance it seems I am paying for everything."

   A. What is a deductible?

   ____

   ____

   ____

   B. What is coinsurance?

   ____

   ____

   ____

   C. What is a copay?

   ____

   ____

   ____

© 2017 Cengage Learning. All Rights Reserved. May not be scanned, copied or duplicated, or posted to a publicly accessible website, in whole or in part.

CHAPTER 23

Performance Improvement and Customer Service

LEARNING OBJECTIVES

Studying and applying the material in this chapter will help you to:

- Understand the components used in determining quality of care.
- Explain what is meant by quality improvement.
- Identify the internal and external customers in a health care setting.
- Describe the steps in working with unhappy customers.
- Describe the characteristics of constructive criticism.
- Discuss how a health care worker can view destructive criticism in a constructive manner.

VOCABULARY REVIEW

Definitions

Write the definition of each of the following words or terms.

1. advocate

____

____

____

2. constructive criticism

____

____

____

© 2017 Cengage Learning. All Rights Reserved. May not be scanned, copied or duplicated, or posted to a publicly accessible website, in whole or in part.

3. external customers

____

____

____

4. internal customers

____

____

____

5. quality improvement

____

____

____

6. utilization review (UR)

____

____

____

CHAPTER REVIEW

True/False

Indicate whether the following statements are true (T) or false (F).

_____ 1. Health care workers must ask themselves what they can do to best meet the needs of the organization, their coworkers, and patients.

_____ 2. When the term *customer* is used, it refers to both internal and external customers.

_____ 3. Outside suppliers of medical and pharmaceutical supplies are considered external customers.

_____ 4. Education would be considered a prevention service.

_____ 5. When a patient evaluates the service received, it is not just the outcome that is important, but the entire experience.

_____ 6. Most facilities have stopped using customer satisfaction surveys as it is more important to look at patient outcomes.

_____ 7. Each health care professional is responsible for patient satisfaction.

_____ 8. Satisfaction is an objective perception.

_____ 9. When people take pride in their work, they will work harder and more cooperatively than they will if they feel that others are being overly critical.

_____ 10. Criticism should not be given to coworkers as it breaks down the working relationship.

© 2017 Cengage Learning. All Rights Reserved. May not be scanned, copied or duplicated, or posted to a publicly accessible website, in whole or in part.

True/False Rewrite

Please rewrite the bold part of the sentence to make the statement true.

1. With the advent of modern health care practices, **it is relatively easy to find the balance between maintaining high-quality patient care and controlling costs**.

2. Spending more on health care **results in better quality of care**.

3. The Centers for Medicare and Medicaid Services (CMS) **impacts only those patients who are on Medicare or Medicaid**.

4. Utilization review (UR) is **a data-collection-only organization**.

5. Patients are an example of an **internal** customer.

6. External customers are those **who work in the health care industry**.

7. **Inpatient services** include nursing homes and assisted living.

8. Illnesses and injuries requiring continuous acute care are considered **emergency and urgent care services**.

© 2017 Cengage Learning. All Rights Reserved. May not be scanned, copied or duplicated, or posted to a publicly accessible website, in whole or in part.

9. Lawsuits are **primarily based on medical errors**.

____

____

____

10. When working with an unhappy customer, **it is best to postpone the conversation until the customer cools off**.

____

____

____

Multiple Choice

Circle the best answer for each of the following questions. There is only one correct answer to each question.

1. Which country ranks highest in health care expenditures?

   A. United States
   B. France
   C. Canada

2. Which of the following is true about Americans' satisfaction with their health care?

   A. most are satisfied
   B. many are dissatisfied
   C. few are dissatisfied

3. Who performs the UR services?

   A. peer review group or public agency
   B. board of directors
   C. governmental agencies

4. What are the UR criteria based upon?

   A. on the money available for patient care
   B. mutual agreement with providers
   C. protocols, benchmarks, or other data

5. Which of the following is true about a Quality Improvement Organization (QIO)?

   A. CMS contracts with one organization in each county
   B. they are private, mostly not-for-profit organizations
   C. they are staffed primarily by lay public

6. What is the first step when working with unhappy customers?

   A. call the supervisor
   B. identify the problem
   C. explain to the customer why it happened

© 2017 Cengage Learning. All Rights Reserved. May not be scanned, copied or duplicated, or posted to a publicly accessible website, in whole or in part.

7. What is the second step when working with unhappy customers?

   A. seek resolution
   B. clarify what the problem is
   C. assure the customer that the person responsible will be reprimanded

8. What is the last step when working with unhappy customers?

   A. tell the customer it won't happen again
   B. apologize profusely
   C. verify satisfaction

9. What is constructive criticism based on?

   A. clarifying the lines of authority
   B. making sure others are quickly corrected
   C. optimism

10. Which of the following is a technique that can be used when giving constructive criticism?

    A. sandwich
    B. telling it like it is
    C. honesty above all else

Short Answer

Read each question. Think about the information presented in the text, and then answer each question.

1. What are the two primary questions that need to be asked when discussing how to improve the quality of care and raise patient satisfaction?

   ____
   ____
   ____

2. What are three factors to consider when trying to measure quality of care?

   ____
   ____
   ____

3. What are the shortcomings of the factors listed in question #2?

   ____
   ____
   ____

4. In health care, the goal is 100% correct care with no errors. Is this realistic? What are the possible consequences if not obtained?

   ____
   ____
   ____

© 2017 Cengage Learning. All Rights Reserved. May not be scanned, copied or duplicated, or posted to a publicly accessible website, in whole or in part.

5. What is the process involved in quality improvement?

____

____

____

6. Who is Centers for Medicare and Medicaid Services (CMS)?

____

____

____

7. Why was CMS designed?

____

____

____

8. What does the CMS require of all health care facilities?

____

____

____

9. The CMS requires all health care facilities to establish a QAPI program that demonstrates a commitment to the goal of ensuring high-quality and cost-effective care. What does the abbreviation QAPI stand for?

____

____

____

10. What are the three primary areas to examine when evaluating a health care facility for quality improvement?

____

____

____

11. What does it mean to serve as a patient advocate?

____

____

____

© 2017 Cengage Learning. All Rights Reserved. May not be scanned, copied or duplicated, or posted to a publicly accessible website, in whole or in part.

Critical Thinking Scenarios

Read each scenario. Think about the information presented in the text, and then answer each question.

1. Ms. Jerkins is furious when a coworker arrives late from lunch. The patients are upset as they are still waiting for services.

   A. What impact is the employee who is late having on the facility?

   ____

   ____

   ____

   B. Should Ms. Jenkins speak to her coworker? If so, when?

   ____

   ____

   ____

   C. What is the difference between constructive and destructive criticism?

   ____

   ____

   ____

2. Mrs. Tomlison calls and states her husband is having chest pain, nausea, and some difficulty breathing. She requests an appointment at the clinic to see his primary care provider.

   A. Should she be given an appointment as requested?

   ____

   ____

   ____

   B. What level of care does the clinic provide?

   ____

   ____

   ____

   C. What level of care does the patient need in this case?

   ____

   ____

   ____

© 2017 Cengage Learning. All Rights Reserved. May not be scanned, copied or duplicated, or posted to a publicly accessible website, in whole or in part.

UNIT 9
Securing and Maintaining Employment

© 2017 Cengage Learning. All Rights Reserved. May not be scanned, copied or duplicated, or posted to a publicly accessible website, in whole or in part.

CHAPTER 24

Job Leads and the Resume

LEARNING OBJECTIVES

Studying and applying the material in this chapter will help you to:

- Develop an inventory of your employment skills and personal traits that are of value to an employer.
- Identify your workplace preferences.
- Describe ways to get organized for the job search.
- List the most common sources of job leads and explain how to use each one effectively.
- Describe the sections of a resume.
- Describe the contents and purpose of chronological and functional resumes.
- List the characteristics of an effective resume.
- Create a resume that highlights your qualifications and encourages employers to interview you.
- Explain the purpose of cover letters.
- Write effective cover letters to accompany your resume.

VOCABULARY REVIEW

Matching

Match the following terms with their correct definitions.

_____	1. chronological resume	A.	emphasizes professional qualifications rather than work history
_____	2. cover letter	B.	emphasizes work experience
_____	3. functional resume	C.	personal characteristics
_____	4. objective	D.	job goal
_____	5. resume	E.	introductory document
_____	6. traits	F.	summary of personal and professional qualifications

© 2017 Cengage Learning. All Rights Reserved. May not be scanned, copied or duplicated, or posted to a publicly accessible website, in whole or in part.

Word Fill

Complete the following sentences by filling in the missing words.

networking cold calling career service centers joblines

1. Schools provide __________________ to help graduates obtain employment.
2. __________________ takes some confidence, but it can be an effective way to discover unadvertised job openings.
3. Recorded information on __________________ enables job seekers to learn about openings at a specific facility.
4. Connecting with other people through __________________ has helped many job seekers start successful careers.

CHAPTER REVIEW

Identification

Place an "X" in front of the sections of a resume that are optional.

_____ 1. special skills

_____ 2. awards and honors

_____ 3. heading

_____ 4. membership in professional organizations

_____ 5. introduction

_____ 6. work history

_____ 7. hobbies and special interests

_____ 8. volunteer work

_____ 9. summary of qualifications

_____ 10. education

True/False Rewrite

Please rewrite the bold part of the sentence to make the statement true.

1. Career professionals recommend that job seekers spend about **10 hours** a week on their job search.

   ____

   ____

   ____

2. **Most** job seekers who post their resumes on the Internet receive multiple job offers as a result.

   ____

   ____

   ____

© 2017 Cengage Learning. All Rights Reserved. May not be scanned, copied or duplicated, or posted to a publicly accessible website, in whole or in part.

3. When seeking a first-time job, your personal preferences should be a **low priority**.

____

____

____

4. A good way to determine what kind of salary you need to earn is to estimate what you spend in **one month**.

____

____

____

5. **Few** students find employment by seeking help from their schools' career services department.

____

____

____

6. If your school schedules an interview for you, but the position doesn't sound interesting, it is **acceptable** to not attend the interview.

____

____

____

7. The reason for attending a job fair is to **interview with as many employers as possible**.

____

____

____

8. Today's most effective way to obtain a job is to **post one's resume on the Internet**.

____

____

____

9. In most cases, a **chronological** resume is the best choice for recent graduates who have no previous health care experience.

____

____

____

10. The purpose of a resume is to convince an employer to **hire you**.

____

____

____

© 2017 Cengage Learning. All Rights Reserved. May not be scanned, copied or duplicated, or posted to a publicly accessible website, in whole or in part.

Multiple Choice

Circle the best answer for each of the following questions. There is only one correct answer to each question.

1. If an announcement for a job states "no calls," it is recommended that you ________.

   A. not call because calling shows your inability to follow instructions
   B. call anyway because this shows you are motivated
   C. not consider this job because the employer does not seem serious

2. The first step when starting your job search is to ________.

   A. consider all the qualifications you have to offer an employer
   B. prepare an outline for your resume
   C. ask the career services staff at your school for assistance

3. The purpose of The Riley Guide at www.rileyguide.com is to ________.

   A. give applicants an opportunity to post their resumes
   B. provide links to health care employers
   C. provide links to websites on all types of career and employment topics

4. Jason plans to use the Internet to make his resume available for employers. Which of the following websites would most likely result in an interview for Jason?

   A. a national general resume-posting site
   B. a health care resume-posting site
   C. a local health care facility's website

5. Prior to enrolling in a nursing program, Liz worked as a preschool teacher. Her best choice would be a ________ resume.

   A. chronological
   B. functional
   C. professional

6. A cover letter should be included with your resume ________.

   A. any time you submit it to an employer
   B. in response to an unadvertised position
   C. when a cover letter is requested

7. Which of the following information should be included in your resume?

   A. your marital status
   B. your telephone number
   C. the statement "references available"

8. Which of the following would best fit in the qualifications section of a resume for a graduate seeking a position as a physical therapist assistant?

   A. earned a 3.7/4.0 grade point average in my physical therapist courses
   B. taught exercise classes at a senior center for 3 years
   C. clinical internship at Get Strong Physical Therapy Clinic, Eugene, Oregon

© 2017 Cengage Learning. All Rights Reserved. May not be scanned, copied or duplicated, or posted to a publicly accessible website, in whole or in part.

Short Answer

Read each question. Think about the information presented in the text, and then answer each question.

1. What are nine factors you should consider when thinking about the type of facility in which you want to work?

___

___

___

2. List six categories of expenses you should consider when calculating your basic living expenses.

___

___

___

3. Why is it important to have an appropriate message on your answering machine or service?

___

___

___

4. What is Career One Stop?

___

___

___

5. What are three types of networking contacts that job seekers can develop?

___

___

___

6. List five ways you can use the Internet in your job search.

___

___

___

7. If you decide to post your resume on the Internet, what information should never be included on the resume?

___

___

___

© 2017 Cengage Learning. All Rights Reserved. May not be scanned, copied or duplicated, or posted to a publicly accessible website, in whole or in part.

8. Why is it recommended that learners write their own resumes rather than having them prepared by a resume service?

____

____

____

9. Why are employment experts advising that job applicants consider not placing their employment objective in their resume?

____

____

____

10. How should your resume be altered if it will be electronically scanned by an employer?

____

____

____

Critical Thinking Scenarios

Read each scenario. Think about the information presented in the text, and then answer each question.

1. Angie has just completed her medical coder course and is eager to get to work. However, she is feeling a little overwhelmed by the job search and is not sure about the best way to find good job leads.

   A. Who should Angie contact first to get started finding leads?

   ____

   ____

   ____

   B. What kinds of websites would likely be most helpful?

   ____

   ____

   ____

   C. What is the web address for the U.S. Department of Labor's website for job hunters?

   ____

   ____

   ____

© 2017 Cengage Learning. All Rights Reserved. May not be scanned, copied or duplicated, or posted to a publicly accessible website, in whole or in part.

2. Andy entered community college directly from high school and has little work experience in any field other than a part-time job in a supermarket. He has almost completed his EMT training and is starting to put together his resume.

   A. Which type of resume would be the best for Andy? Explain why.

   ____

   ____

   ____

   B. Which section, after the heading and objective, should he place at the beginning of his resume? Explain why.

   ____

   ____

   ____

© 2017 Cengage Learning. All Rights Reserved. May not be scanned, copied or duplicated, or posted to a publicly accessible website, in whole or in part.

CHAPTER 25

Interview, Portfolio, and Application

LEARNING OBJECTIVES

Studying and applying the material in this chapter will help you to:

- Explain the purpose of the job interview.
- Describe how to obtain background information about employers and health care organizations.
- Create examples to illustrate your employment qualifications.
- Prepare appropriate questions to ask at interviews.
- Anticipate and prepare for questions that may be asked at interviews.
- Describe ways to handle illegal questions asked by employers.
- Demonstrate successful interview behavior and appearance.
- Identify references who will support your job search efforts.
- Create a reference list to give to potential employers.
- Build a professional portfolio to provide evidence of your job skills and qualifications.
- Explain what actions to take after an interview to increase your chances of being hired.
- Explain how to accept and reject job offers.

© 2017 Cengage Learning. All Rights Reserved. May not be scanned, copied or duplicated, or posted to a publicly accessible website, in whole or in part.

VOCABULARY REVIEW

Word Fill

Complete the following sentences by filling in the missing words.

job interview	references	illegal questions	situational question
letter of recommendation	portfolio	reference list	behavioral questions

1. Employers now use ________________ to learn how applicants have handled workplace problems in the past.
2. Employers cannot use information obtained from ________________ to make hiring decisions.
3. The purpose of the ________________ is for employers and applicants to learn about each other.
4. It is a good idea to ask for a/an ________________ whenever you leave a job on good terms.
5. A collection of documents you might use at an interview to support your qualifications is called a/an ________________.
6. Be sure to ask your ________________ for permission before giving their names to prospective employers.
7. Your ________________ contains the names and contact information of people who will vouch for your qualifications.
8. An example of a/an ________________ is, "Tell me about how you would handle working with a rude patient."

CHAPTER REVIEW

True/False

Indicate whether the following statements are true (T) or false (F).

____ 1. Job applicants can best present themselves at interviews by being modest.

____ 2. The interview is a good time to ask for a job description of the position for which you are applying.

____ 3. Applicants should prepare questions in advance to ask at an interview.

____ 4. Asking about benefits and vacation days is appropriate at the first interview if you are interested in the job.

____ 5. If an employer asks you about your weaknesses, it is best to state that you really can't think of any.

____ 6. Your appearance makes an important statement about you as a professional.

____ 7. Perfumes that most people find pleasant can be offensive to people who are ill.

____ 8. Some employers are becoming more accepting of tattoos and piercings on health care professionals.

© 2017 Cengage Learning. All Rights Reserved. May not be scanned, copied or duplicated, or posted to a publicly accessible website, in whole or in part.

_____ 9. Your portfolio should be sent along with your resume.

_____ 10. Listening at an interview is just as important as speaking well.

_____ 11. It is illegal for employers to require new hires to be tested for drugs.

_____ 12. If you are offered a job that you decide you don't want, it is recommended that you explain to the employer why you are not accepting it.

Multiple Choice

Circle the best answer for each of the following questions. There is only one correct answer to each question.

1. Which of the following best describes the purpose of a job interview?
   A. a time for employers to ask questions and find out if applicants fill their requirements
   B. gives applicants a chance to learn about a job
   C. gives applicants and employers an opportunity to learn about each other

2. Which action on the part of applicants is most likely to help them do well at job interviews?
   A. participate in mock interviews
   B. write a great resume
   C. put together a good portfolio

3. Angie has failed to get hired after attending several interviews. Which of the following is most likely the cause of her failure to get a job?
   A. does not have previous health care work experience
   B. did not graduate at the top of her class
   C. does not sell herself well

4. Which of the following is the best reason for creating a personal inventory of skills and traits?
   A. build your confidence for interviewing and asking for a job
   B. give you examples to demonstrate and support your skills
   C. have a written list to give to employers

5. Which of the following questions would be most appropriate for an applicant to ask at an interview for a job in a small, single-physician office?
   A. "What are the opportunities for promotion?"
   B. "What type of orientation would I receive?"
   C. "How much would I be earning after a year of work?"

6. The best answers to behavioral questions consist of a/an ____________________.
   A. description of a past experience
   B. short answer that is to the point
   C. explanation of how you have improved

7. Which of the following is an example of an illegal question?
   A. "Where are your parents from?"
   B. "Can you work nights?"
   C. "How do you handle stressful situations?"

© 2017 Cengage Learning. All Rights Reserved. May not be scanned, copied or duplicated, or posted to a publicly accessible website, in whole or in part.

8. John was fired from his last job for taking too many breaks. Which is his best response if a prospective employer asks if he has ever been fired?
   A. "No, I haven't."
   B. "Yes, my last boss really didn't like me."
   C. "Yes. I used to take too many smoke breaks. I have since quit smoking and started an exercise program, so this is no longer a problem for me."
9. Jan, a single mother with three school-age children, is interviewing for a job she really wants. If the employer asks her if she has young children, it would be best for her to state, "________________."
   A. "That question is illegal."
   B. "I don't have to answer questions about my family."
   C. "I have children and have arranged for very dependable child-care."
10. Which of the following would be the best person to ask to write you a letter of recommendation?
   A. a family friend who has known you since childhood
   B. the supervisor at your extern site
   C. your dentist

Matching

Match the following types of interview questions with the example that best illustrates it.

_____	1. general employment question	A. Is Friday casual dress day?
_____	2. illegal question	B. Have you ever been arrested?
_____	3. behavioral question	C. Can you tell me why you've had so many jobs?
_____	4. appropriate question to ask employer	D. Why do you want to work here?
_____	5. question to avoid asking employer	E. Tell me the steps you would take to clean up a blood spill.
_____	6. health care question	F. Tell me about a conflict you've had with a coworker and how you resolved it.
_____	7. question to answer honestly	G. What is a typical day like for someone in this position?

Short Answer

Read each question. Think about the information presented in the text, and then answer each question.

1. Why do some employers find the interview process to be a stressful experience?

____

____

____

© 2017 Cengage Learning. All Rights Reserved. May not be scanned, copied or duplicated, or posted to a publicly accessible website, in whole or in part.

2. What are three reasons for learning about an employer before attending an interview?

3. List four sources you might use to learn about prospective employers.

4. What is the best way to demonstrate to an employer that you have the skills needed for the job?

5. When answering general questions such as, "Tell me about yourself," what should you be sure to include in your answer?

6. List five items that would be appropriate to include in your portfolio.

7. What three actions should you take when you meet the person who will interview you?

8. Why is it important for a job applicant to be courteous with the receptionist when arriving for an interview?

9. Under what circumstances should you send a thank-you note following an interview?

© 2017 Cengage Learning. All Rights Reserved. May not be scanned, copied or duplicated, or posted to a publicly accessible website, in whole or in part.

10. What are eight guidelines for correctly filling out an employment application?

Critical Thinking Scenarios

Read each scenario. Think about the information presented in the text, and then answer each question.

1. Chad is interviewing for a job as a physical therapist assistant. The employer asks what part of town he lives in.
   A. Is this an appropriate question for the employer to ask? Explain.

   B. Why might the employer ask this question?

   C. How should Chad respond?

2. Kayla interviewed for a job in health information management at the clinic where her own doctor practices. This was a job she really wanted and she felt she interviewed well. However, she just received word that she did not get the job.
   A. What are possible reasons why Kayla was not offered this job?

   B. What should Kayla do now?

   C. What should Kayla do if she attends many interviews and fails to receive a job offer?

© 2017 Cengage Learning. All Rights Reserved. May not be scanned, copied or duplicated, or posted to a publicly accessible website, in whole or in part.

CHAPTER 26

Successful Employment Strategies

LEARNING OBJECTIVES

Studying and applying the material in this chapter will help you to:

- Identify important information that new employees should learn about the facility in which they work.
- Explain the importance of understanding the facility's policies and procedures.
- Explain the purpose of the probationary period.
- Identify seven behaviors that contribute to professional success.
- List and describe the major laws that affect hiring and employment practices.
- Explain the meaning of a grievance and how it should be handled.
- Explain the meaning of sexual harassment and the actions to take if it occurs.
- Describe a typical performance evaluation.
- Identify the steps to take when leaving a job voluntarily.
- Describe ways to cope with being fired from a job.
- List activities that promote professional development of the health care professional.

VOCABULARY REVIEW

Matching 1

Match the following terms with their correct definitions.

_____	1. chain of command	A.	correct way to perform a task
_____	2. grievance	B.	plans and methods to ensure safety
_____	3. minimum wage	C.	least amount of pay legally allowed
_____	4. policy	D.	change that enables a disabled person to function in the workplace
_____	5. procedure	E.	levels of authority and reporting
_____	6. reasonable accommodation	F.	unwelcome and/or offensive actions
_____	7. risk management	G.	established rule or course of action
_____	8. sexual harassment	H.	formal complaint

© 2017 Cengage Learning. All Rights Reserved. May not be scanned, copied or duplicated, or posted to a publicly accessible website, in whole or in part.

Word Fill

Complete the following sentences by filling in the missing words.

employee manual	integrity	professional development	job description
role model	probationary period	performance evaluation	mentor
team			

1. Having a ________________ to give you information and encouragement can contribute to a successful career.
2. Review your ________________ carefully so you know what your duties are.
3. The ________________ gives the employer and employee a chance to see how things are working out for each of them.
4. ________________ includes learning activities that help you improve your career knowledge and performance.
5. New hires are likely to be part of a/an ________________ of professionals working together.
6. A/an ________________ is a person who serves as a positive example of professionalism.
7. Check the ________________ to learn about the organization in which you work.
8. Going through a/an ________________ helps both you and your employer track your progress.
9. Honesty and morality are signs of ________________, an important quality for health care professionals.

CHAPTER REVIEW

True/False

Indicate whether the following statements are true (T) or false (F).

_____ 1. Failure to follow safety policies can be grounds for dismissal from a job.

_____ 2. In many states, employees can be dismissed for any reason during the probationary period.

_____ 3. Completing their tasks satisfactorily is all that most employers expect of an employee.

_____ 4. Having many points of view, as from the members of a work team, makes completing projects an inefficient and difficult process.

_____ 5. New employees are not really expected to make significant contributions to workplace teams.

_____ 6. Knowing when to ask for help is an important work skill.

_____ 7. It is generally necessary to do more than the minimum job requirements to achieve career success.

_____ 8. A good strategy at work is to avoid problems whenever possible.

© 2017 Cengage Learning. All Rights Reserved. May not be scanned, copied or duplicated, or posted to a publicly accessible website, in whole or in part.

_____ 9. Performance evaluations do not always include a salary review.

_____ 10. Employees should be prepared to argue and defend themselves if they receive low ratings in their performance evaluation.

_____ 11. Employees have the right to view the contents of their personnel files.

_____ 12. When leaving a job, it is recommended that you state your reasons for quitting, including complaints that were not resolved.

_____ 13. It is usually advisable to find a new job before leaving the present one.

_____ 14. Failure to follow standard practices can be a cause for dismissal.

_____ 15. One week's notice is usually adequate when leaving a job.

Multiple Choice

Circle the best answer for each of the following questions. There is only one correct answer to each question.

1. Which is the most important reason for following a facility's policies and procedures?

   A. They give consistency to the facility's operations.
   B. They may be legally required.
   C. They give your supervisor a way to measure your performance.

2. Information about paid holidays would most likely be found in a/an ________________.

   A. employee manual
   B. handbook of procedures
   C. job description

3. Providing a worker with a desk chair that has extra back support is an example of a ________________.

   A. working condition
   B. reasonable accommodation
   C. grievance

4. The main purpose of the probationary period is to ________________.

   A. determine if the employee should receive a raise
   B. teach the employee needed job skills
   C. give the employer an opportunity to evaluate the employee

5. Which of the following is the best example of an employee demonstrating integrity?

   A. Amy always greets patients with a smile and friendly greeting.
   B. John forgot to make an important note on a patient chart and he tells the physician as soon as he realizes his mistake.
   C. Sarah takes extra time to explain procedures to patients to help them feel more comfortable and less anxious.

6. Which of the following behaviors best demonstrates loyalty to the employer?

   A. Dan discusses problems he's having with the employer with his coworkers.
   B. Liz speaks with her supervisor privately about the problems she's having at work.
   C. Lauren complains about her supervisor to her husband after work.

© 2017 Cengage Learning. All Rights Reserved. May not be scanned, copied or duplicated, or posted to a publicly accessible website, in whole or in part.

7. Observing the chain of command means to ________________.
   A. warn your supervisor's boss about problems in your department
   B. report problems to your supervisor
   C. share problems with your coworkers
8. When would it acceptable to make personal phone calls during work hours?
   A. If you have a family emergency
   B. When you don't have work to do
   C. It is never acceptable
9. If you tend to procrastinate when faced with a large task, it is recommended that you ________________.
   A. start with the easiest part first
   B. get started and push to do as much as possible
   C. break the task down into manageable parts
10. If you have a personal conflict with a team member, it is best to ________________.
    A. keep the matter to yourself
    B. discuss the matter with the team member in private
    C. bring the matter into the open at a team meeting

Matching 2

Match the following laws with the examples that best illustrate them.

____	1. Title VII of 1964 Civil Rights Act	A.	BeWell Health Clinic cannot refuse to hire applicants because they are not Christian.
____	2. Family Medical Leave Act	B.	Happy Home Health cannot hire aides who do not have the legal right to work in the United States.
____	3. Americans with Disabilities Act	C.	Good Care Hospital cannot deny employment to a qualified medical coder because she has a hearing impairment.
____	4. Equal Pay Act of 1963	D.	Dr. Cromwell must pay his medical assistant no less than what his state requires.
____	5. minimum wage laws	E.	Ashley wants to take a few weeks off after the birth of her child.
____	6. Civil Rights Act of 1964	F.	Ellie advises her supervisor that his unwanted comments about her "sexy" appearance are violating her legal rights.
____	7. Occupational Safety and Health Act	G.	Good Care Hospital provides free hepatitis B immunizations for all employees who provide direct patient care.
____	8. Immigration Reform Act	H.	The Caring Clinic must pay Carol and Tim, both medical assistants with four years of experience, the same salary.

© 2017 Cengage Learning. All Rights Reserved. May not be scanned, copied or duplicated, or posted to a publicly accessible website, in whole or in part.

Completion

Use the words in the list to complete the following statements:

enthusiasm	policy	role model	quality control
flexibility	professional development	supervisor	networking
performance evaluation	sexual harassment		

1. Proofreading a report written for work and correcting any errors is an example of ________________.
2. Signs of ________________ are being passionate about and interested in your work.
3. Identifying a/an ________________ at your first job can help you learn how to be a true professional in your occupation.
4. Telling off-color jokes in the presence of someone who finds them offensive is a form of ________________.
5. Employees can improve their work performance by actively participating with their supervisor during their ________________.
6. When quitting a job, you should first advise your ________________.
7. Many workplaces have a/an ________________ that requires a supervisor to observe a fired employee as he or she packs up personal belongings.
8. An important part of ________________ is setting goals and learning new skills.
9. ________________ should be carried out throughout your career both for your own benefit and that of others.
10. Health care professionals should demonstrate ________________ by responding well to changing conditions in the workplace.

Critical Thinking Scenarios

Read each scenario. Think about the information presented in the text, and then answer each question.

1. Roberto has been working at LiveWell Center for three years. During the past six months, he has been feeling dissatisfied with his job and wonders if he should look for a new one.

   A. In making his decision, what should Roberto do first?

   ____

   ____

   ____

   B. What factors should he consider when comparing his current job with other possibilities?

   ____

   ____

   ____

© 2017 Cengage Learning. All Rights Reserved. May not be scanned, copied or duplicated, or posted to a publicly accessible website, in whole or in part.

C. If Roberto decides to leave his job, how should he proceed?

____

____

____

2. Andrea has been working at her first job as a medical sonographer for two weeks. Her position had been vacant for some time and the supervisor did not have a lot of time to give her an orientation to the facility.

A. What are sources of information that Andrea might use to learn more about the facility and what she is expected to do?

____

____

____

B. Why is it important for her to pay special attention to the facility's risk management policies?

____

____

____

C. As a new employee, when should Andrea expect to have her first employment evaluation?

____

____

____

© 2017 Cengage Learning. All Rights Reserved. May not be scanned, copied or duplicated, or posted to a publicly accessible website, in whole or in part.

Procedure Assessments

© 2017 Cengage Learning. All Rights Reserved. May not be scanned, copied or duplicated, or posted to a publicly accessible website, in whole or in part.

Name: ______________________ Date: __________ Score: __________

Procedure Assessment 10-1: Handwashing

Task: Performing proper handwashing technique

Standard: Complete the skill in 5 minutes with a minimum of 70% within three attempts.

Scoring: Divide points earned by total possible points. Failure to perform any of the following critical steps will result in an unsatisfactory overall score.

Time Began ______________ Time Ended ______________

No.	Steps	Points	Check #1	Check #2	Check #3
1.	Turn faucet on using a clean, dry paper towel.	10			
2.	Run warm water over hands and wrists.	10			
3.	Do not lean against the sink, and avoid splashing clothing with water.	10			
4.	Keep hands lower than arms during procedure, and keep fingertips pointing downward.	10			
5.	Apply liquid soap to hands.	10			
6.	Scrub palms in a circular motion while clasping hands together.	10			
7.	Scrub wrists 1 to 2 inches above the hands by encircling one wrist with the other hand; then repeat for other wrist.	10			
8.	Scrub the back of each hand with a circular motion by cupping one hand over the other.	10			
9.	Scrub between the fingers with a back-and-forth motion by interlacing fingers.	10			
10.	Scrub each individual finger and clean under the nails with a cuticle stick, a brush, or a fingernail on the other hand, or by rubbing it against the palm of the other hand.	10			
11.	Scrub hands for at least 2 minutes.	10			
12.	Rinse each hand thoroughly with running water from the wrists down to the fingertips.	10			

© 2017 Cengage Learning. All Rights Reserved. May not be scanned, copied or duplicated, or posted to a publicly accessible website, in whole or in part.

No.	Steps	Points	Check #1	Check #2	Check #3
13.	Dry thoroughly with a disposable towel(s).	10			
14.	Use another dry towel to turn off the faucet handle.	10			
15.	Clean sink area using dry towels, being careful not to recontaminate hands by touching any surfaces.	10			
16.	Use lotion if desired.	0			
	Student's Total Points				
	Points Possible	150			
	Final Score (Student's Total Points/ Possible Points)				

Instructor's/Evaluator's Comments and Suggestions:

____

____

____

____

Evaluator's Signature: ______________________ **Date:** ____________

© 2017 Cengage Learning. All Rights Reserved. May not be scanned, copied or duplicated, or posted to a publicly accessible website, in whole or in part.

Name: ________________________ Date: __________ Score: __________

Procedure Assessment 10-2: Nonsterile Gloves

Task: Applying and removing nonsterile gloves

Standard: Complete the skill in 5 minutes with a minimum of 70% within three attempts.

Scoring: Divide points earned by total possible points. Failure to perform any of the following critical steps will result in an unsatisfactory overall score.

Time Began ____________________ Time Ended ____________________

No.	Steps	Points	Check #1	Check #2	Check #3
1.	Use proper handwashing technique before applying gloves.	10			
2.	Remove appropriate-sized clean gloves from the box and apply (touch only the gloves you will be using when removing them from the dispenser).	10			
3.	To remove gloves: Grasp the outside of one glove at the palm with the other gloved hand; pull the glove down and turn it inside out while removing it.	10			
4.	Hold the removed glove in the palm of the remaining gloved hand.	10			
5.	Take the ungloved hand and slide it under the cuff of the remaining glove and push the glove off (the first glove is now inside the second glove that was removed).	10			
6.	Discard the gloves in an appropriate container according to facility policy.	10			
7.	Wash hands immediately after removing gloves.	10			
	Student's Total Points				
	Points Possible	70			
	Final Score (Student's Total Points/ Possible Points)				

© 2017 Cengage Learning. All Rights Reserved. May not be scanned, copied or duplicated, or posted to a publicly accessible website, in whole or in part.

Instructor's/Evaluator's Comments and Suggestions:

____

____

____

____

Evaluator's Signature: ______________________________ **Date:** ____________

© 2017 Cengage Learning. All Rights Reserved. May not be scanned, copied or duplicated, or posted to a publicly accessible website, in whole or in part.

Name: ____________________ Date: __________ Score: __________

Procedure Assessment 10-3: PPE (Personal Protective Equipment)

Task: Applying and removing PPE

Standard: Complete the skill in 10 minutes with a minimum of 70% within three attempts.

Scoring: Divide points earned by total possible points. Failure to perform any of the following critical steps will result in an unsatisfactory overall score.

Time Began ____________ Time Ended ____________

No.	Steps	Points	Check #1	Check #2	Check #3
1.	Use proper handwashing technique before applying PPE.	10			
2.	Put on cap, mask, protective eyewear, and gown. No specific sequence of applying these items is required.	10			
3.	To apply gown: Put on the gown by placing your hands inside the shoulders. Slip your fingers inside the neckband to tie the gown at the neck. Overlap the back edges of the gown so your uniform is completely covered before tying the waist ties.	10			
4.	Apply gloves last: Remove appropriate-sized clean gloves from the box and apply. Touch only the gloves you will be using when removing them from the dispenser. Pull the cuffs over the sleeves of the gown to create a seal.	10			
5.	Remove PPE: Untie the waist ties of the gown. Remove contaminated gloves. Wash hands. Remove cap and protective eyewear gently.	10			

© 2017 Cengage Learning. All Rights Reserved. May not be scanned, copied or duplicated, or posted to a publicly accessible website, in whole or in part.

No.	Steps	Points	Check #1	Check #2	Check #3
6.	To remove gown: Untie the neck tie of the gown. Slip the fingers of one hand under the cuff of the opposite arm and pull the gown down until it covers the hand. Using the gown-covered hand, grasp the outside of the gown on the opposite arm, and pull the gown down until it covers the hand. Both hands are now inside the gown and can be used to grasp the outside of the gown. Use your covered hands to grasp the gown at the shoulders and turn the gown inside out (contaminated side on the inside) as you remove it. Roll it up and place in appropriate container. Remove the mask. Hold the mask by the strings to discard it.	10			
7.	Wash hands.	10			
	Student's Total Points				
	Points Possible	70			
	Final Score (Student's Total Points/ Possible Points)				

Instructor's/Evaluator's Comments and Suggestions:

____

____

____

____

Evaluator's Signature: ______________________ **Date:** ____________

© 2017 Cengage Learning. All Rights Reserved. May not be scanned, copied or duplicated, or posted to a publicly accessible website, in whole or in part.

Name: ______________________ Date: ________ Score: ________

Procedure Assessment 10-4: Sterile Gloves

Task: Applying sterile gloves

Standard: Complete the skill in 5 minutes with a minimum of 70% within three attempts.

Scoring: Divide points earned by total possible points. Failure to perform any of the following critical steps will result in an unsatisfactory overall score.

Time Began ______________ Time Ended ______________

No.	Steps	Points	Check #1	Check #2	Check #3
1.	Use proper handwashing technique before applying sterile gloves.	10			
2.	Inspect glove package for tears or stains and do not use if present.	10			
3.	Place package of gloves on a clean, dry, flat surface above waist level.	10			
4.	Open sterile gloves by pulling back on the tabs without touching the sterile inner border.	10			
5.	The gloves should be opened with the cuffs toward you, the palms up, and the thumbs pointing outward. If the gloves are not positioned properly, turn the package around, being careful not to reach over the sterile area or touch the inner surface of the gloves.	10			
6.	Pick up the first glove by grasping the glove on the top edge of the folded-down cuff. Do not drag or dangle the fingers over any nonsterile area.	10			
7.	Maintain the grasp on the cuff, insert your other hand, and gently pull the glove on by the cuff. Always hold the hands above the waist and away from the body with palms up.	10			
8.	Slip the gloved fingers under the cuff of the second glove to lift it from the package and insert the other hand into the glove.	10			
9.	Pull the glove on and adjust the glove into position, being careful not to touch the skin with the gloved hands.	10			

© 2017 Cengage Learning. All Rights Reserved. May not be scanned, copied or duplicated, or posted to a publicly accessible website, in whole or in part.

No.	Steps	Points	Check #1	Check #2	Check #3
10.	Turn the cuffs up by manipulating only the sterile surface of the gloves (go under the folded cuffs, pull out slightly, and turn cuffs over and up).	10			
11.	Check the gloves for tears, holes, and imperfections.	10			
	Student's Total Points				
	Points Possible	110			
	Final Score (Student's Total Points/ Possible Points)				

Instructor's/Evaluator's Comments and Suggestions:

____

____

____

____

Evaluator's Signature: ______________________ **Date:** ______________

© 2017 Cengage Learning. All Rights Reserved. May not be scanned, copied or duplicated, or posted to a publicly accessible website, in whole or in part.

Name: ____________________ Date: ________ Score: ________

Procedure Assessment 20-1a: Temperature—Oral

Task: Obtaining an oral temperature

Standard: Complete the skill in 5 minutes with a minimum of 70% within three attempts.

Scoring: Divide points earned by total possible points. Failure to perform any of the following critical steps will result in an unsatisfactory overall score.

Work Documentation: Document findings in patient's chart.

Time Began ____________ Time Ended ____________

No.	Steps	Points	Check #1	Check #2	Check #3
1.	Use proper handwashing technique before taking a temperature. Apply gloves if needed.	10			
2.	Verify that the patient has not taken any food or fluid by mouth, smoked, or chewed gum in the last 30 minutes	10			
3.	Clean with alcohol and when dry, apply temperature probe sheath.	10			
4.	Ask the patient to open mouth.	10			
5.	Place the thermometer under the tongue on either side, as close to the midline as possible.	10			
6.	Instruct patient to close lips around thermometer but to not bite down on it.	10			
7.	Leave it in place until unit signals a final reading.	10			
8.	Remove thermometer and read digital display.	10			
9.	Record your findings.	10			
10.	Remove temperature probe sheath and dispose of properly. Clean thermometer with alcohol.	10			
	Student's Total Points				
	Points Possible	100			
	Final Score (Student's Total Points/ Possible Points)				

© 2017 Cengage Learning. All Rights Reserved. May not be scanned, copied or duplicated, or posted to a publicly accessible website, in whole or in part.

CHART FINDINGS

____

____

Instructor's/Evaluator's Comments and Suggestions:

____

____

____

____

Evaluator's Signature: ______________________ **Date:** ____________

© 2017 Cengage Learning. All Rights Reserved. May not be scanned, copied or duplicated, or posted to a publicly accessible website, in whole or in part.

Name: ______________________ Date: __________ Score: __________

Procedure Assessment 20-1b: Temperature—Axillary

Task: Obtaining an axillary temperature

Standard: Complete the skill in 5 minutes with a minimum of 70% within three attempts.

Scoring: Divide points earned by total possible points. Failure to perform any of the following critical steps will result in an unsatisfactory overall score.

Work Documentation: Document findings in patient's chart.

Time Began __________________ Time Ended __________________

No.	Steps	Points	Check #1	Check #2	Check #3
1.	Use proper handwashing technique before taking a temperature. Apply gloves if needed.	10			
2.	Clean with alcohol and when dry, apply temperature probe sheath.	10			
3.	Remove clothing from patient's shoulder and arm.	10			
4.	Ensure that axillary area is dry, wiping with dry towel if necessary.	10			
5.	Place thermometer in the center of the armpit and place arm across the abdomen and close to side of body.	10			
6.	Leave it in place until unit signals a final reading.	10			
7.	Remove thermometer and read digital display.	10			
8.	Record your findings.	10			
9.	Remove temperature probe sheath and dispose of properly. Clean thermometer with alcohol.	10			
	Student's Total Points				
	Points Possible	90			
	Final Score (Student's Total Points/ Possible Points)				

© 2017 Cengage Learning. All Rights Reserved. May not be scanned, copied or duplicated, or posted to a publicly accessible website, in whole or in part.

CHART FINDINGS

____

____

Instructor's/Evaluator's Comments and Suggestions:

____

____

____

____

Evaluator's Signature: ______________________ **Date:** ____________

© 2017 Cengage Learning. All Rights Reserved. May not be scanned, copied or duplicated, or posted to a publicly accessible website, in whole or in part.

Name: ______________________ Date: __________ Score: __________

Procedure Assessment 20-1c: Temperature—Rectal

Task: Obtaining a rectal temperature

Standard: Complete the skill in 5 minutes with a minimum of 70% within three attempts.

Scoring: Divide points earned by total possible points. Failure to perform any of the following critical steps will result in an unsatisfactory overall score.

Work Documentation: Document findings in patient's chart.

Time Began ______________ Time Ended ______________

No.	Steps	Points	Check #1	Check #2	Check #3
1.	Use proper handwashing technique before taking a temperature. Apply gloves.	10			
2.	Clean with alcohol and when dry, apply temperature probe sheath.	10			
3.	Ensure that adults are in a side-lying position with top leg flexed forward.	10			
4.	Lubricate the thermometer.	10			
5.	Insert the thermometer into the rectum (1 inch for children, and 1½ inches for adults).	10			
6.	Hold tip of thermometer while in place.	10			
7.	Leave it in place until unit signals a final reading.	10			
8.	Remove thermometer and read digital display.	10			
9.	Record your findings.	10			
10.	Remove temperature probe sheath and dispose of properly. Clean thermometer with alcohol.	10			
	Student's Total Points				
	Points Possible	100			
	Final Score (Student's Total Points/ Possible Points)				

© 2017 Cengage Learning. All Rights Reserved. May not be scanned, copied or duplicated, or posted to a publicly accessible website, in whole or in part.

CHART FINDINGS

____

____

Instructor's/Evaluator's Comments and Suggestions:

____

____

____

____

Evaluator's Signature: ______________________________ **Date:** ______________

© 2017 Cengage Learning. All Rights Reserved. May not be scanned, copied or duplicated, or posted to a publicly accessible website, in whole or in part.

Name: ______________________ Date: __________ Score: __________

Procedure Assessment 20-1d: Temperature—Aural (Tympanic)

Task: Obtaining an aural (tympanic) temperature

Standard: Complete the skill in 5 minutes with a minimum of 70% within three attempts.

Scoring: Divide points earned by total possible points. Failure to perform any of the following critical steps will result in an unsatisfactory overall score.

Work Documentation: Document findings in patient's chart.

Time Began __________ Time Ended __________

No.	Steps	Points	Check #1	Check #2	Check #3
1.	Use proper handwashing technique before taking a temperature.	10			
2.	Place disposable probe on the thermometer.	10			
3.	Stabilize the patient's head.	10			
4.	In children younger than 1 year, gently pull the ear straight back; in children older than 1 year and adults, pull the ear back and up.	10			
5.	Insert the probe into ear canal until you obtain seal.	10			
6.	Remove thermometer and read digital display.	10			
7.	Record your findings.	10			
8.	Properly dispose of probe.	10			
	Student's Total Points				
	Points Possible	80			
	Final Score (Student's Total Points/ Possible Points)				

CHART FINDINGS

____

____

Instructor's/Evaluator's Comments and Suggestions:

____

____

____

____

Evaluator's Signature: ______________________ **Date:** __________

© 2017 Cengage Learning. All Rights Reserved. May not be scanned, copied or duplicated, or posted to a publicly accessible website, in whole or in part.

Name: ______________________ Date: __________ Score: __________

Procedure Assessment 20-1e: Temperature—Temporal Artery

Task: Obtaining a temporal artery temperature

Standard: Complete the skill in 5 minutes with a minimum of 70% within three attempts.

Scoring: Divide points earned by total possible points. Failure to perform any of the following critical steps will result in an unsatisfactory overall score.

Work Documentation: Document findings in patient's chart.

Time Began ______________ Time Ended ______________

No.	Steps	Points	Check #1	Check #2	Check #3
1.	Use proper handwashing technique before taking a temperature.	10			
2.	Clean probe with alcohol and let dry.	10			
3.	Remove perspiration from forehead, remove hat, push back hair from forehead.	10			
4.	Center the probe on the forehead (midline), press the scan button, and slowly move it across forehead to the temple area hair line.	10			
5.	Record your findings.	10			
6.	Clean probe with alcohol, let dry, and return to holder.	10			
	Student's Total Points				
	Points Possible	60			
	Final Score (Student's Total Points/ Possible Points)				

CHART FINDINGS

____

____

Instructor's/Evaluator's Comments and Suggestions:

____

____

____

____

Evaluator's Signature: ______________________ **Date:** ______________

© 2017 Cengage Learning. All Rights Reserved. May not be scanned, copied or duplicated, or posted to a publicly accessible website, in whole or in part.

Name: ______________________ Date: __________ Score: __________

Procedure Assessments 20-2 and 20-4: Radial Pulse and Respirations (the procedure for taking respirations is included along with taking the pulse because, since the respiratory rate can be consciously altered, it is important that the patient not know when you are counting the respirations)

Task: Obtaining a radial pulse and respirations

Standard: Complete the skill in 5 minutes with a minimum of 70% within three attempts.

Scoring: Divide points earned by total possible points. Failure to perform any of the following critical steps will result in an unsatisfactory overall score.

Work Documentation: Document findings in patient's chart.

Time Began ____________ Time Ended ____________

No.	Steps	Points	Check #1	Check #2	Check #3
1.	Use proper handwashing technique before taking the radial pulse and respirations.	10			
2.	Locate the radial pulse by gently but firmly pressing on the thumb side of the wrist until an indented area is felt; use two to three fingers to feel the pulse.	10			
3.	Place the patient's hand on his or her chest.	10			
4.	Count the pulsations you feel in a 60-second period and note any variances from normal in rhythm or pulse volume.	10			
5.	When you complete the procedure, leave your fingers on the pulse, and count the respirations in a 60-second period noting any variances from normal in rhythm or respiratory effort.	10			
6.	Record your findings.	10			
	Student's Total Points				
	Points Possible	60			
	Final Score (Student's Total Points/ Possible Points)				

© 2017 Cengage Learning. All Rights Reserved. May not be scanned, copied or duplicated, or posted to a publicly accessible website, in whole or in part.

CHART FINDINGS

____

____

Instructor's/Evaluator's Comments and Suggestions:

____

____

____

____

Evaluator's Signature: ______________________ **Date:** ____________

© 2017 Cengage Learning. All Rights Reserved. May not be scanned, copied or duplicated, or posted to a publicly accessible website, in whole or in part.

Name: ____________________ Date: ________ Score: ________

Procedure Assessment 20-3 and 20-4: Apical Pulse and Respirations (the procedure for taking respirations is included along with taking the pulse because, since the respiratory rate can be consciously altered, it is important that the patient not know when you are counting the respirations)

Task: Obtaining an apical pulse and respirations

Standard: Complete the skill in 5 minutes with a minimum of 70% within three attempts.

Scoring: Divide points earned by total possible points. Failure to perform any of the following critical steps will result in an unsatisfactory overall score.

Work Documentation: Document findings in patient's chart.

Time Began ____________ Time Ended ____________

No.	Steps	Points	Check #1	Check #2	Check #3
1.	Use proper handwashing technique before taking the apical pulse and respirations.	10			
2.	Wipe the earpieces and diaphragm of stethoscope with alcohol wipes, and inspect the stethoscope prior to use.	10			
3.	Verify that the diaphragm side is where the sound will be heard.	10			
4.	If the diaphragm is cold to the touch, rub it against your clothing or hand until it is warm.	10			
5.	Place earpieces into your ears, with the earpieces pointing forward.	10			
6.	Place the diaphragm of the stethoscope directly on the skin, over the apex of the heart, and hold it with gentle but firm pressure.	10			
7.	Instruct the patient to breathe normally.	10			
8.	Count the beats you hear in a 60-second period noting any variances from normal in rhythm or pulse volume.	10			

© 2017 Cengage Learning. All Rights Reserved. May not be scanned, copied or duplicated, or posted to a publicly accessible website, in whole or in part.

No.	Steps	Points	Check #1	Check #2	Check #3
9.	When you are done, leave the stethoscope in place and count the respirations in a 60-second period noting any variances from normal in rhythm or respiratory effort.	10			
10.	Record your findings.	10			
	Student's Total Points				
	Points Possible	100			
	Final Score (Student's Total Points/ Possible Points)				

CHART FINDINGS

____

____

Instructor's/Evaluator's Comments and Suggestions:

____

____

____

____

Evaluator's Signature: ______________________ **Date:** ______________

© 2017 Cengage Learning. All Rights Reserved. May not be scanned, copied or duplicated, or posted to a publicly accessible website, in whole or in part.

Name: ______________________ Date: __________ Score: __________

Procedure Assessment 20-5: Manual Blood Pressure

Task: Obtain a manual blood pressure reading

Standard: Complete the skill in 5 minutes with a minimum of 70% within three attempts.

Scoring: Divide points earned by total possible points. Failure to perform any of the following critical steps will result in an unsatisfactory overall score.

Work Documentation: Document findings in patient's chart.

Time Began ______________ Time Ended ______________

No.	Steps	Points	Check #1	Check #2	Check #3
1.	Use proper handwashing technique before taking the manual blood pressure.	10			
2.	Verify that the cuff is the correct size for the patient and that the valve is closed to allow for inflation of bladder.	10			
3.	Place the patient in a relaxed lying or sitting position, remove the clothing from the arm, and position the arm at heart level. Instruct the patient not to talk during the procedure.	10			
4.	Locate the pulse of the brachial artery in the inner aspect of the antecubital space, and place the arrows on the cuff over this area.	10			
5.	Place your fingers on the radial artery and inflate the cuff until you can no longer feel the pulse. Note the reading and add 30 to it.	10			
6.	Deflate the cuff by opening the screw. Wait at least 30 seconds.	10			
7.	Place the stethoscope in your ears and place the diaphragm over the brachial artery. Press gently.	10			
8.	Close the screw and inflate the cuff to the predetermined amount from Step 5.	10			
9.	Slowly release the screw so the cuff deflates evenly (about 2 mm Hg at a time), and listen for the first sound of the pulse returning to the brachial artery. Make a mental note of the reading.	10			

© 2017 Cengage Learning. All Rights Reserved. May not be scanned, copied or duplicated, or posted to a publicly accessible website, in whole or in part.

No.	Steps	Points	Check #1	Check #2	Check #3
10.	Continue allowing the cuff to deflate until you no longer hear any sounds from the brachial artery. Make a mental note of the reading.	10			
11.	Continue to listen for any return of sounds from the brachial artery for an additional 20 to 30 mm Hg.	10			
12.	Open the screw completely and let the cuff deflate rapidly.	10			
13.	Remove the stethoscope from your ears and the cuff from the patient's arm and immediately record your results in even numbers only (manual blood pressure) along with which arm was used.	10			
14.	If you are unsure of the blood pressure readings and want to recheck it, use the other arm or wait several minutes before using the same arm.	10			
	Student's Total Points				
	Points Possible	140			
	Final Score (Student's Total Points/ Possible Points)				

CHART FINDINGS

____

____

Instructor's/Evaluator's Comments and Suggestions:

____

____

____

____

Evaluator's Signature: ______________________ **Date:** ____________

© 2017 Cengage Learning. All Rights Reserved. May not be scanned, copied or duplicated, or posted to a publicly accessible website, in whole or in part.

Name: ______________________ Date: __________ Score: __________

Procedure Assessment 21-la: Allergic Reactions—Mild to Moderate

Task: Giving first aid for mild to moderate allergic reactions

Standard: Complete the skill in 5 minutes with a minimum of 70% within three attempts.

Scoring: Divide points earned by total possible points. Failure to perform any of the following critical steps will result in an unsatisfactory overall score.

Work Documentation: Document findings in patient's chart.

Time Began __________________ Time Ended __________________

No.	Steps	Points	Check #1	Check #2	Check #3
1.	Use proper handwashing technique and apply PPE as appropriate before giving first aid.	10			
2.	Be calm and reassuring in approach to victim.	10			
3.	If there is an itchy rash, apply anti-itch lotion (e.g., calamine lotion) and cool compresses.	10			
4.	Try to determine the source of the allergic reaction.	10			
5.	A physician may recommend an over-the-counter medication (e.g., diphenhydramine).	10			
6.	Call EMS if the condition worsens	10			
	Student's Total Points				
	Points Possible	60			
	Final Score (Student's Total Points/ Possible Points)				

CHART FINDINGS

____

____

Instructor's/Evaluator's Comments and Suggestions:

____

____

____

____

Evaluator's Signature: ______________________ **Date:** __________

© 2017 Cengage Learning. All Rights Reserved. May not be scanned, copied or duplicated, or posted to a publicly accessible website, in whole or in part.

Name: ______________________ Date: __________ Score: __________

Procedure Assessment 21-1b: Allergic Reactions—Severe

Task: Giving first aid for severe allergic reactions

Standard: Complete the skill in 5 minutes with a minimum of 70% within three attempts.

Scoring: Divide points earned by total possible points. Failure to perform any of the following critical steps will result in an unsatisfactory overall score.

Work Documentation: Document findings in patient's chart.

Time Began ______________ Time Ended ______________

No.	Steps	Points	Check #1	Check #2	Check #3
1.	Use proper handwashing technique and apply PPE as appropriate before giving first aid.	10			
2.	Be calm and reassuring in approach to victim.	10			
3.	Call EMS.	10			
4.	If the victim has emergency allergy medication, help him or her administer it.	10			
5.	Do not give the victim anything by mouth if he or she is having difficulty breathing.	10			
6.	Do not place a pillow under the victim's head.	10			
	Student's Total Points				
	Points Possible	60			
	Final Score (Student's Total Points/ Possible Points)				

CHART FINDINGS

____

____

Instructor's/Evaluator's Comments and Suggestions:

____

____

____

____

Evaluator's Signature: ______________________ **Date:** ______________

© 2017 Cengage Learning. All Rights Reserved. May not be scanned, copied or duplicated, or posted to a publicly accessible website, in whole or in part.

Name: ______________________ Date: __________ Score: __________

Procedure Assessment 21-1c: Allergic Reactions—Bites and Stings

Task: Giving first aid for bites and stings

Standard: Complete the skill in 10 minutes with a minimum of 70% within three attempts.

Scoring: Divide points earned by total possible points. Failure to perform any of the following critical steps will result in an unsatisfactory overall score.

Work Documentation: Document findings in patient's chart.

Time Began ______________ Time Ended ______________

No.	Steps	Points	Check #1	Check #2	Check #3
1.	Use proper handwashing technique and apply PPE as appropriate before giving first aid.	10			
2.	Be calm and reassuring in approach to victim.	10			
3.	Try to identify what bit or stung the victim.	10			
4.	Kill it if there is no risk to the rescuer, and keep it for identification.	10			
5.	If there is a stinger: Remove it by scraping it with your fingernail or a credit card.	10			
6.	If there is a tick: Do not forcibly remove a tick; instead suffocate it by covering it with a heavy oil (e.g., Vaseline, mineral oil), wait 30 minutes, then carefully remove it with tweezers, placing them as close to the mouth parts as possible (if all parts are not removed, seek medical attention).	10			
7.	If it is poisonous: Call EMS immediately if a poisonous spider, scorpion, or snake has bitten the victim.	10			
8.	If an allergic reaction occurs, treat it as noted for allergic reactions (Procedures 21-1a and 21-1b).	10			
9.	Stay with the victim for at least an hour.	10			

© 2017 Cengage Learning. All Rights Reserved. May not be scanned, copied or duplicated, or posted to a publicly accessible website, in whole or in part.

No.	Steps	Points	Check #1	Check #2	Check #3
10.	Clean the area with soap and water and apply antiseptic ointment.	10			
11.	Remove any confining clothing or jewelry.	10			
12.	Apply a cold compress.	10			
13.	Have the victim lie still and keep the bite area below heart level.	10			
14.	Do not apply a tourniquet.	10			
15.	Consult with a physician to determine if any additional preventive measures should be taken.	10			
16.	Instruct the victim to observe for infection (e.g., increased pain, redness, or swelling; discharge from the site, swollen glands, fever, flu-like symptoms, or red streaks coming from site) and get medical help immediately if symptoms occur.	10			
	Student's Total Points				
	Points Possible	160			
	Final Score (Student's Total Points/ Possible Points)				

CHART FINDINGS

____

____

Instructor's/Evaluator's Comments and Suggestions:

____

____

____

____

Evaluator's Signature: ______________________ **Date:** __________

© 2017 Cengage Learning. All Rights Reserved. May not be scanned, copied or duplicated, or posted to a publicly accessible website, in whole or in part.

Name: ______________________ Date: __________ Score: __________

Procedure Assessment 21-2a: Bleeding and Wounds—External Bleeding

Task: Giving first aid for external bleeding

Standard: Complete the skill in 5 minutes with a minimum of 70% within three attempts.

Scoring: Divide points earned by total possible points. Failure to perform any of the following critical steps will result in an unsatisfactory overall score.

Work Documentation: Document findings in patient's chart.

Time Began ______________ Time Ended ______________

No.	Steps	Points	Check #1	Check #2	Check #3
1.	Use proper handwashing technique and apply PPE as appropriate before giving first aid.	10			
2.	Be calm and reassuring in approach to victim.	10			
3.	Call EMS if you suspect internal bleeding or if there is heavy external bleeding or other serious injuries.	10			
4.	Apply cold compresses to bruised areas.	10			
5.	If bleeding from the leg or arm, elevate it above heart level (unless contraindicated by neck or back injury, or discomfort).	10			
6.	Do not use a tourniquet.	10			
7.	To stop bleeding, apply direct pressure with a clean cloth or sterile dressing over the area. If the rescuer needs his or her hands free to do additional first aid, a pressure dressing can be applied to decrease the bleeding.	10			
8.	When the dressing becomes soaked with blood, do not remove it; instead place the new dressing on top. Do not look under the dressing to see if the bleeding has stopped.	10			
9.	Do not apply pressure over an embedded object, the eye, or on a head injury if a skull fracture is suspected.	10			

© 2017 Cengage Learning. All Rights Reserved. May not be scanned, copied or duplicated, or posted to a publicly accessible website, in whole or in part.

No.	Steps	Points	Check #1	Check #2	Check #3
10.	If bleeding from an arm or leg does not stop after 15 minutes of direct pressure, then use pressure-point bleeding control.	10			
	Student's Total Points				
	Points Possible	100			
	Final Score (Student's Total Points/ Possible Points)				

CHART FINDINGS

____

____

Instructor's/Evaluator's Comments and Suggestions:

____

____

____

____

Evaluator's Signature: ______________________________ **Date:** ______________

© 2017 Cengage Learning. All Rights Reserved. May not be scanned, copied or duplicated, or posted to a publicly accessible website, in whole or in part.

Name: ________________________ Date: ________ Score: ________

Procedure Assessment 21-2b: Bleeding and Wounds—Internal Bleeding

Task: Giving first aid for internal bleeding

Standard: Complete the skill in 5 minutes with a minimum of 70% within three attempts.

Scoring: Divide points earned by total possible points. Failure to perform any of the following critical steps will result in an unsatisfactory overall score.

Work Documentation: Document findings in patient's chart.

Time Began ________________ Time Ended ________________

No.	Steps	Points	Check #1	Check #2	Check #3
1.	Use proper handwashing technique and apply PPE as appropriate before giving first aid.	10			
2.	Be calm and reassuring in approach to victim.	10			
3.	Call EMS.	10			
4.	Do not give the victim anything to eat or drink.	10			
5.	Place the victim on his or her back and elevate the knees with a pillow or blanket if there is abdominal discomfort.	10			
6.	Keep the victim still and treat him or her for shock as needed.	10			
7.	Stay with victim until medical assistance arrives.	10			
	Student's Total Points				
	Points Possible	70			
	Final Score (Student's Total Points/ Possible Points)				

© 2017 Cengage Learning. All Rights Reserved. May not be scanned, copied or duplicated, or posted to a publicly accessible website, in whole or in part.

CHART FINDINGS

____

____

Instructor's/Evaluator's Comments and Suggestions:

____

____

____

____

Evaluator's Signature: ______________________________ **Date:** ______________

© 2017 Cengage Learning. All Rights Reserved. May not be scanned, copied or duplicated, or posted to a publicly accessible website, in whole or in part.

Name: ______________________ Date: __________ Score: __________

Procedure Assessment 21-2c: Bleeding and Wounds—Wounds

Task: Giving first aid for wounds, including sucking wounds

Standard: Complete the skill in 5 minutes with a minimum of 70% within three attempts.

Scoring: Divide points earned by total possible points. Failure to perform any of the following critical steps will result in an unsatisfactory overall score.

Work Documentation: Document findings in patient's chart.

Time Began ____________________ Time Ended ____________________

No.	Steps	Points	Check #1	Check #2	Check #3
1.	Use proper handwashing technique and apply PPE as appropriate before giving first aid.	10			
2.	Be calm and reassuring in approach to victim.	10			
3.	Do not try to clean a large wound or remove any embedded objects.	10			
4.	Remove any obvious loose debris from the wound.	10			
5.	If an object is protruding from the body, do not remove it.	10			
6.	Sucking Wound: If the chest or neck has been punctured or if there is an object protruding from the chest or neck, note if there is any bubbling from the wound. If so, this is called a sucking wound, and it needs to be sealed as soon as possible.	10			
7.	With a sucking wound, apply an airtight dressing (e.g., plastic wrap, tin foil, plastic bag, or other nonporous material) over the site. If you do not have nonporous material, you can use a regular gauze pad or clean cloth coated with petroleum jelly (e.g., Vaseline).	10			
8.	When applying an airtight dressing, leave one edge untaped or unsealed.	10			
9.	Do not move the patient unless absolutely necessary.	10			

© 2017 Cengage Learning. All Rights Reserved. May not be scanned, copied or duplicated, or posted to a publicly accessible website, in whole or in part.

No.	Steps	Points	Check #1	Check #2	Check #3
10.	Do not give the patient anything by mouth.	10			
	Student's Total Points				
	Points Possible	100			
	Final Score (Student's Total Points/ Possible Points)				

CHART FINDINGS

____

____

Instructor's/Evaluator's Comments and Suggestions:

____

____

____

____

Evaluator's Signature: ______________________ **Date:** ______________

© 2017 Cengage Learning. All Rights Reserved. May not be scanned, copied or duplicated, or posted to a publicly accessible website, in whole or in part.

Name: ______________________ Date: __________ Score: __________

Procedure Assessment 21-2d: Bleeding and Wounds—Amputation

Task: Giving first aid for amputation

Standard: Complete the skill in 5 minutes with a minimum of 70% within three attempts.

Scoring: Divide points earned by total possible points. Failure to perform any of the following critical steps will result in an unsatisfactory overall score.

Work Documentation: Document findings in patient's chart.

Time Began ____________________ Time Ended ____________________

No.	Steps	Points	Check #1	Check #2	Check #3
1.	Use proper handwashing technique and apply PPE as appropriate before giving first aid.	10			
2.	Be calm and reassuring in approach to victim.	10			
3.	If an amputation of a body part occurs, save the severed part.	10			
4.	After giving the appropriate first aid to the victim, try to locate the part if it is not in the immediate area.	10			
5.	Once the body part is found, rinse it off, wrap it in a moistened cloth, and place it in a plastic bag or other container.	10			
6.	If ice is available, place the bag in a container with ice and water. Do not place the part directly on ice.	10			
7.	Write the name of the patient and the time of the accident on the container with the body part.	10			
8.	Make sure the amputated body part remains with the victim when he or she is transported to the hospital.	10			
	Student's Total Points				
	Points Possible	80			
	Final Score (Student's Total Points/ Possible Points)				

© 2017 Cengage Learning. All Rights Reserved. May not be scanned, copied or duplicated, or posted to a publicly accessible website, in whole or in part.

CHART FINDINGS

____

____

Instructor's/Evaluator's Comments and Suggestions:

____

____

____

____

Evaluator's Signature: ____________________ **Date:** ____________

© 2017 Cengage Learning. All Rights Reserved. May not be scanned, copied or duplicated, or posted to a publicly accessible website, in whole or in part.

Name: ______________________ Date: ________ Score: ________

Procedure Assessment 21-3a: Bone, Joint, and Muscle Injuries—Fractures and Joint Dislocations

Task: Giving first aid for fractures and joint dislocations

Standard: Complete the skill in 5 minutes with a minimum of 70% within three attempts.

Scoring: Divide points earned by total possible points. Failure to perform any of the following critical steps will result in an unsatisfactory overall score.

Work Documentation: Document findings in patient's chart.

Time Began ______________ Time Ended ______________

No.	Steps	Points	Check #1	Check #2	Check #3
1.	Use proper handwashing technique and apply PPE as appropriate before giving first aid.	10			
2.	Be calm and reassuring in approach to victim.	10			
3.	Do not move the victim until the affected limb is immobilized unless there is no other option.	10			
4.	Immobilize the broken bone or dislocated joint using a splint.	10			
5.	Do not attempt to realign a misshapen bone or joint. Do not test for function.	10			
6.	Do not give anything by mouth.	10			
7.	If there is an open fracture, cover it with a dressing prior to immobilizing the area. Do not wash or attempt to remove anything from the area.	10			
8.	When immobilizing an area, leave it in the position you found it and make sure that the area above and below is extra well-supported, so the injured area is immobilized.	10			
9.	Check for circulation below the injury to ensure that the splint is not too tight.	10			
	Student's Total Points				
	Points Possible	90			
	Final Score (Student's Total Points/ Possible Points)				

© 2017 Cengage Learning. All Rights Reserved. May not be scanned, copied or duplicated, or posted to a publicly accessible website, in whole or in part.

CHART FINDINGS

____

____

Instructor's/Evaluator's Comments and Suggestions:

____

____

____

____

Evaluator's Signature: ______________________________ **Date:** ______________

© 2017 Cengage Learning. All Rights Reserved. May not be scanned, copied or duplicated, or posted to a publicly accessible website, in whole or in part.

Name: ______________________ Date: __________ Score: __________

Procedure Assessment 21-3b: Bone, Joint, and Muscle Injuries—Strains and Sprains

Task: Giving first aid for strains and sprains

Standard: Complete the skill in 5 minutes with a minimum of 70% within three attempts.

Scoring: Divide points earned by total possible points. Failure to perform any of the following critical steps will result in an unsatisfactory overall score.

Work Documentation: Document findings in patient's chart.

Time Began __________ Time Ended __________

No.	Steps	Points	Check #1	Check #2	Check #3
1.	Use proper handwashing technique and apply PPE as appropriate before giving first aid.	10			
2.	Be calm and reassuring in approach to victim.	10			
3.	Remove any constricting clothing or jewelry.	10			
4.	Apply cold compresses as soon as possible and repeat every 3–4 hours for 15–20 minutes.	10			
5.	Do not place ice directly on the skin.	10			
6.	Elevate the limb.	10			
7.	Contact a physician if the pain is severe, if there is loss of function or impairment of circulation below injury, or if the area is misshapen.	10			
8.	A physician may also recommend an over-the-counter anti-inflammatory medication.	10			
9.	Rest the injured area for at least 24 hours. Do not use the injured area if pain occurs with movement.	10			
10.	If there is no improvement, seek medical assistance.	10			

© 2017 Cengage Learning. All Rights Reserved. May not be scanned, copied or duplicated, or posted to a publicly accessible website, in whole or in part.

No.	Steps	Points	Check #1	Check #2	Check #3
	Student's Total Points				
	Points Possible	100			
	Final Score (Student's Total Points/ Possible Points)				

CHART FINDINGS

____

____

Instructor's/Evaluator's Comments and Suggestions:

____

____

____

____

Evaluator's Signature: ______________________________ **Date:** ________________

© 2017 Cengage Learning. All Rights Reserved. May not be scanned, copied or duplicated, or posted to a publicly accessible website, in whole or in part.

Name: ______________________ Date: __________ Score: __________

Procedure Assessment 21-4a: Facial Injuries—Eye

Task: Giving first aid for eye injuries

Standard: Complete the skill in 5 minutes with a minimum of 70% within three attempts.

Scoring: Divide points earned by total possible points. Failure to perform any of the following critical steps will result in an unsatisfactory overall score.

Work Documentation: Document findings in patient's chart.

Time Began ______________ Time Ended ______________

No.	Steps	Points	Check #1	Check #2	Check #3
1.	Use proper handwashing technique and apply PPE as appropriate before giving first aid.	10			
2.	Be calm and reassuring in approach to victim.	10			
3.	Do not press on the eye or allow the victim to rub the eyes.	10			
4.	If a foreign object is irritating the eye, flush the eye with a large amount of water.	10			
5.	Do not use cotton swabs (e.g., Q-tips) or any instruments (e.g., tweezers) to try to remove objects from eye.	10			
6.	If the object is not flushed out and is embedded, do not attempt to remove it; instead cover both eyes with a dressing and await medical assistance.	10			
7.	If there has been a blow to the eye, lay the victim flat, cover both eyes, and call for medical assistance.	10			
8.	If a "black eye" is forming, apply a cold compress to the area.	10			
	Student's Total Points				
	Points Possible	80			
	Final Score (Student's Total Points/ Possible Points)				

© 2017 Cengage Learning. All Rights Reserved. May not be scanned, copied or duplicated, or posted to a publicly accessible website, in whole or in part.

CHART FINDINGS

____

____

Instructor's/Evaluator's Comments and Suggestions:

____

____

____

____

Evaluator's Signature: ______________________ **Date:** ____________

© 2017 Cengage Learning. All Rights Reserved. May not be scanned, copied or duplicated, or posted to a publicly accessible website, in whole or in part.

Name: ______________________ Date: __________ Score: __________

Procedure Assessment 21-4b: Facial Injuries—Ear

Task: Giving first aid for ear injuries

Standard: Complete the skill in 5 minutes with a minimum of 70% within three attempts.

Scoring: Divide points earned by total possible points. Failure to perform any of the following critical steps will result in an unsatisfactory overall score.

Work Documentation: Document findings in patient's chart.

Time Began ____________ Time Ended ____________

No.	Steps	Points	Check #1	Check #2	Check #3
1.	Use proper handwashing technique and apply PPE as appropriate before giving first aid.	10			
2.	Be calm and reassuring in approach to victim.	10			
3.	Do not block bleeding or drainage from the ear. If possible, lay the victim on his or her side with the injured ear down.	10			
4.	Do not attempt to clean inside the ear.	10			
5.	If an object is in the ear and clearly visible, place the victim's injured ear downward and gently wiggle the object with tweezers.	10			
6.	Do not attempt to remove an object that is not visible. Seek medical assistance.	10			
7.	If ruptured eardrum is suspected, place a dressing over the ear. Seek medical assistance.	10			
8.	If an insect is in the ear, do not allow the victim to poke a finger into the ear. Have the victim hold his or her head with the ear pointing up.	10			

© 2017 Cengage Learning. All Rights Reserved. May not be scanned, copied or duplicated, or posted to a publicly accessible website, in whole or in part.

No.	Steps	Points	Check #1	Check #2	Check #3
9.	If medical assistance is not immediately available, the victim is very uncomfortable, and you are sure it is only an insect, place several drops of room-temperature oil into the ear (e.g., cooking oil, baby oil, mineral oil). Seek medical assistance.	10			
	Student's Total Points				
	Points Possible	90			
	Final Score (Student's Total Points/ Possible Points)				

CHART FINDINGS

____

____

Instructor's/Evaluator's Comments and Suggestions:

____

____

____

____

Evaluator's Signature: ______________________ **Date:** ____________

© 2017 Cengage Learning. All Rights Reserved. May not be scanned, copied or duplicated, or posted to a publicly accessible website, in whole or in part.

Name: ______________________ Date: __________ Score: __________

Procedure Assessment 21-4c: Facial Injuries—Nose

Task: Giving first aid for nose injuries

Standard: Complete the skill in 5 minutes with a minimum of 70% within three attempts.

Scoring: Divide points earned by total possible points. Failure to perform any of the following critical steps will result in an unsatisfactory overall score.

Work Documentation: Document findings in patient's chart.

Time Began ______________ Time Ended ______________

No.	Steps	Points	Check #1	Check #2	Check #3
1.	Use proper handwashing technique and apply PPE as appropriate before giving first aid.	10			
2.	Be calm and reassuring in approach to victim.	10			
3.	If there is an object lodged in the nostril, attempt to remove it by having the victim hold the other nostril and blow out the nostril with the object, or have the victim sniff some pepper to induce a sneeze. If this does not work, get medical help.	10			
4.	Do not put anything into the nostril to try to grab hold of the object.	10			
5.	Instruct the victim to breathe through the mouth and not inhale through the nostril.	10			
6.	If the nose may be broken, have the victim sit down, lean forward, and apply a cold compress.	10			
7.	Do not attempt to straighten a broken nose, but seek medical assistance.	10			

© 2017 Cengage Learning. All Rights Reserved. May not be scanned, copied or duplicated, or posted to a publicly accessible website, in whole or in part.

No.	Steps	Points	Check #1	Check #2	Check #3
8.	If the nose is not broken, attempt to stop the bleeding by instructing the victim to sit down and lean forward while applying pressure on the soft part of the nose. Maintain the pressure for at least 15 minutes, then release. If there's still bleeding, repeat the procedure for 15 more minutes. Then, if it has not stopped, seek medical assistance.	10			
	Student's Total Points				
	Points Possible	80			
	Final Score (Student's Total Points/ Possible Points)				

CHART FINDINGS

___

___

Instructor's/Evaluator's Comments and Suggestions:

___

___

___

___

Evaluator's Signature: ______________________ **Date:** ______________

© 2017 Cengage Learning. All Rights Reserved. May not be scanned, copied or duplicated, or posted to a publicly accessible website, in whole or in part.

Name: ______________________ Date: __________ Score: __________

Procedure Assessment 21-5a: Burns—Heat

Task: Giving first aid for heat burns

Standard: Complete the skill in 5 minutes with a minimum of 70% within three attempts.

Scoring: Divide points earned by total possible points. Failure to perform any of the following critical steps will result in an unsatisfactory overall score.

Work Documentation: Document findings in patient's chart.

Time Began ____________ Time Ended ____________

No.	Steps	Points	Check #1	Check #2	Check #3
1.	Use proper handwashing technique and apply PPE as appropriate before giving first aid.	10			
2.	Be calm and reassuring in approach to victim.	10			
3.	Extinguish the fire (i.e., if the victim's clothing is on fire).	10			
4.	Move the victim to a well-ventilated area if smoke is present. Move accident victims only when it is necessary to protect them.	10			
5.	When moving victims, maintain their body alignment.	10			
6.	Run cool water over the burned area for several minutes or immerse the area in cool water (use a cool, wet cloth on areas that cannot be immersed and rewet as necessary by pouring additional cool water onto the cloth).	10			
7.	Do not apply ice except on a minor burn, such as a finger burned on the stove.	10			
8.	Remove clothing from the burn area if possible, but if it's stuck to the burn, do not use force.	10			
9.	Do not break blisters.	10			
10.	Cover the burn with a clean, dry cloth (use sterile, nonadhesive dressings if available).	10			

© 2017 Cengage Learning. All Rights Reserved. May not be scanned, copied or duplicated, or posted to a publicly accessible website, in whole or in part.

No.	Steps	Points	Check #1	Check #2	Check #3
11.	Do not apply any ointments to a severe burn.	10			
12.	Apply a bandage loosely.	10			
13.	Do not use cotton as a dressing.	10			
14.	Prevent chilling.	10			
	Student's Total Points				
	Points Possible	140			
	Final Score (Student's Total Points/ Possible Points)				

CHART FINDINGS

____

____

Instructor's/Evaluator's Comments and Suggestions:

____

____

____

____

Evaluator's Signature: ______________________ **Date:** ____________

© 2017 Cengage Learning. All Rights Reserved. May not be scanned, copied or duplicated, or posted to a publicly accessible website, in whole or in part.

Name: ______________________ Date: __________ Score: __________

Procedure Assessment 21-5b: Burns—Radiation

Task: Giving first aid for radiation burns

Standard: Complete the skill in 5 minutes with a minimum of 70% within three attempts.

Scoring: Divide points earned by total possible points. Failure to perform any of the following critical steps will result in an unsatisfactory overall score.

Work Documentation: Document findings in patient's chart.

Time Began __________ Time Ended __________

No.	Steps	Points	Check #1	Check #2	Check #3
1.	Use proper handwashing technique and apply PPE as appropriate before giving first aid.	10			
2.	Be calm and reassuring in approach to victim.	10			
3.	Move the victim so he or she is no longer exposed to the sun.	10			
4.	Run cool water over the burned area for several minutes or immerse the area in cool water (use a cool, wet cloth on areas that cannot be immersed and rewet as necessary by pouring additional cool water onto the cloth).	10			
5.	Do not break blisters.	10			
6.	Cover the burn with a clean, dry cloth (use sterile, nonadhesive dressings if available).	10			
7.	Do not apply any ointments to a severe burn.	10			
8.	Apply a bandage loosely.	10			
9.	Do not use cotton as a dressing.	10			
10.	Prevent chilling.	10			
	Student's Total Points				
	Points Possible	100			
	Final Score (Student's Total Points/ Possible Points)				

© 2017 Cengage Learning. All Rights Reserved. May not be scanned, copied or duplicated, or posted to a publicly accessible website, in whole or in part.

CHART FINDINGS

____

____

Instructor's/Evaluator's Comments and Suggestions:

____

____

____

____

Evaluator's Signature: ______________________ **Date:** ____________

© 2017 Cengage Learning. All Rights Reserved. May not be scanned, copied or duplicated, or posted to a publicly accessible website, in whole or in part.

Name: ______________________ Date: __________ Score: __________

Procedure Assessment 21-5c: Burns—Chemical

Task: Giving first aid for chemical burns

Standard: Complete the skill in 5 minutes with a minimum of 70% within three attempts.

Scoring: Divide points earned by total possible points. Failure to perform any of the following critical steps will result in an unsatisfactory overall score.

Work Documentation: Document findings in patient's chart.

Time Began ______________ Time Ended ______________

No.	Steps	Points	Check #1	Check #2	Check #3
1.	Use proper handwashing technique and apply PPE as appropriate before giving first aid.	10			
2.	Be calm and reassuring in approach to victim.	10			
3.	Prevent any further contact of the victim with the chemical.	10			
4.	Move the victim to a well-ventilated area if fumes are present. Move accident victims only when it is necessary to protect them.	10			
5.	When moving victims, maintain their body alignment.	10			
6.	Flush the burn with large amounts of cool water and continue to do so until EMS arrives.	10			
7.	Always flush away from the body.	10			
8.	If there is any chemical in the eyes, flush them continuously with cool water.	10			
9.	If only one eye is affected, flush from the inner aspect of the eye to the outer.	10			
	Student's Total Points				
	Points Possible	90			
	Final Score (Student's Total Points/ Possible Points)				

© 2017 Cengage Learning. All Rights Reserved. May not be scanned, copied or duplicated, or posted to a publicly accessible website, in whole or in part.

CHART FINDINGS

____

____

Instructor's/Evaluator's Comments and Suggestions:

____

____

____

____

Evaluator's Signature: ______________________________ **Date:** ________________

© 2017 Cengage Learning. All Rights Reserved. May not be scanned, copied or duplicated, or posted to a publicly accessible website, in whole or in part.

Name: ______________________ Date: __________ Score: __________

Procedure Assessment 21-5d: Burns—Electrical

Task: Giving first aid for electrical current burns

Standard: Complete the skill in 5 minutes with a minimum of 70% within three attempts.

Scoring: Divide points earned by total possible points. Failure to perform any of the following critical steps will result in an unsatisfactory overall score.

Work Documentation: Document findings in patient's chart.

Time Began ______________ Time Ended ______________

No.	Steps	Points	Check #1	Check #2	Check #3
1.	Use proper handwashing technique and apply PPE as appropriate before giving first aid.	10			
2.	Be calm and reassuring in approach to victim.	10			
3.	Do not touch the victim if he or she is still in contact with a live electrical wire (have the power turned off first).	10			
4.	Do not cool the burn.	10			
5.	Apply a clean, dry dressing.	10			
6.	Prevent chilling and do not move the victim if possible, because other injuries may be present.	10			
7.	If necessary to move the victim, maintain the victim's body alignment.	10			
	Student's Total Points				
	Points Possible	70			
	Final Score (Student's Total Points/ Possible Points)				

CHART FINDINGS

____

____

Instructor's/Evaluator's Comments and Suggestions:

____

____

____

____

Evaluator's Signature: ______________________ **Date:** ______________

© 2017 Cengage Learning. All Rights Reserved. May not be scanned, copied or duplicated, or posted to a publicly accessible website, in whole or in part.

Name: ______________________________ Date: __________ Score: __________

Procedure Assessment 21-6a: Drug-Related Problems—Overdose

Task: Giving first aid for drug overdose

Standard: Complete the skill in 3 minutes with a minimum of 70% within three attempts.

Scoring: Divide points earned by total possible points. Failure to perform any of the following critical steps will result in an unsatisfactory overall score.

Work Documentation: Document findings in patient's chart.

Time Began ______________ Time Ended ______________

No.	Steps	Points	Check #1	Check #2	Check #3
1.	Use proper handwashing technique and apply PPE as appropriate before giving first aid.	10			
2.	Be calm and reassuring in approach to victim.	10			
3.	Call EMS.	10			
4.	Try to determine what was taken, when, how much, and which route (e.g., oral, inhalation, injection). Be aware that it may have been more than one type or also combined with alcohol or other substances.	10			
5.	If possible, collect samples of the drug and of any vomit for analysis.	10			
	Student's Total Points				
	Points Possible	50			
	Final Score (Student's Total Points/ Possible Points)				

CHART FINDINGS

____

____

Instructor's/Evaluator's Comments and Suggestions:

____

____

____

____

Evaluator's Signature: ______________________ **Date:** ______________

© 2017 Cengage Learning. All Rights Reserved. May not be scanned, copied or duplicated, or posted to a publicly accessible website, in whole or in part.

Name: ______________________ Date: __________ Score: __________

Procedure Assessment 21-6b: Drug-Related Problems—Withdrawal

Task: Giving first aid for withdrawal from addictive drug

Standard: Complete the skill in 3 minutes with a minimum of 70% within three attempts.

Scoring: Divide points earned by total possible points. Failure to perform any of the following critical steps will result in an unsatisfactory overall score.

Work Documentation: Document findings in patient's chart.

Time Began ______________ Time Ended ______________

No.	Steps	Points	Check #1	Check #2	Check #3
1.	Use proper handwashing technique and apply PPE as appropriate before giving first aid.	10			
2.	Be calm and reassuring in approach to victim.	10			
3.	Call EMS.	10			
4.	Try to determine what drug the victim has been taking.	10			
5.	Keep the victim safe and comfortable until medical assistance arrives.	10			
	Student's Total Points				
	Points Possible	50			
	Final Score (Student's Total Points/ Possible Points)				

CHART FINDINGS

____

____

Instructor's/Evaluator's Comments and Suggestions:

____

____

____

____

Evaluator's Signature: ______________________ **Date:** ______________

© 2017 Cengage Learning. All Rights Reserved. May not be scanned, copied or duplicated, or posted to a publicly accessible website, in whole or in part.

Name: ______________________ Date: __________ Score: __________

Procedure Assessment 21-7a: Poisonings—Ingested

Task: Giving first aid for ingested poison

Standard: Complete the skill in 5 minutes with a minimum of 70% within three attempts.

Scoring: Divide points earned by total possible points. Failure to perform any of the following critical steps will result in an unsatisfactory overall score.

Work Documentation: Document findings in patient's chart.

Time Began ______________ Time Ended ______________

No.	Steps	Points	Check #1	Check #2	Check #3
1.	Use proper handwashing technique and apply PPE as appropriate before giving first aid.	10			
2.	Be calm and reassuring in approach to victim.	10			
3.	Do not administer any food, fluids, or home remedies or induce vomiting unless directed to do so by medical personnel.	10			
4.	If the victim does vomit, make sure the vomit is cleared from the mouth.	10			
5.	Save any vomit.	10			
6.	Keep the patient safe and comfortable until help can arrive.	10			
	Student's Total Points				
	Points Possible	60			
	Final Score (Student's Total Points/ Possible Points)				

CHART FINDINGS

____

____

Instructor's/Evaluator's Comments and Suggestions:

____

____

____

____

Evaluator's Signature: ______________________ **Date:** ______________

© 2017 Cengage Learning. All Rights Reserved. May not be scanned, copied or duplicated, or posted to a publicly accessible website, in whole or in part.

Name: ______________________ Date: __________ Score: __________

Procedure Assessment 21-7b: Poisonings—Inhaled

Task: Giving first aid for inhaled poison

Standard: Complete the skill in 5 minutes with a minimum of 70% within three attempts.

Scoring: Divide points earned by total possible points. Failure to perform any of the following critical steps will result in an unsatisfactory overall score.

Work Documentation: Document findings in patient's chart.

Time Began ______________ Time Ended ______________

No.	Steps	Points	Check #1	Check #2	Check #3
1.	Use proper handwashing technique and apply PPE as appropriate before giving first aid.	10			
2.	Be calm and reassuring in approach to victim.	10			
3.	Get the victim into fresh air.	10			
4.	Before entering an environment where poisonous gases may be present, apply protective breathing gear. If no protective breathing gear is available, place a wet cloth over your nose and mouth, and then take several deep breaths of fresh air before entering to remove the victim.	10			
5.	If there is a visible cloud of fumes, keep your head above or below it.	10			
6.	If possible, open windows and doors and turn off any source of fumes.	10			
7.	Do not light any flames or flip any switches.	10			
8.	When the victim is in fresh air, the Poison Control Center or EMS can be called.	10			
9.	The victim should be kept safe and comfortable until help arrives.	10			
	Student's Total Points				
	Points Possible	90			
	Final Score (Student's Total Points/ Possible Points)				

© 2017 Cengage Learning. All Rights Reserved. May not be scanned, copied or duplicated, or posted to a publicly accessible website, in whole or in part.

CHART FINDINGS

____

____

Instructor's/Evaluator's Comments and Suggestions:

____

____

____

____

Evaluator's Signature: ______________________________ **Date:** ______________

© 2017 Cengage Learning. All Rights Reserved. May not be scanned, copied or duplicated, or posted to a publicly accessible website, in whole or in part.

Name: ______________________ Date: __________ Score: __________

Procedure Assessment 21-8a: Temperature-Related Illnesses—Frostbite

Task: Giving first aid for frostbite

Standard: Complete the skill in 5 minutes with a minimum of 70% within three attempts.

Scoring: Divide points earned by total possible points. Failure to perform any of the following critical steps will result in an unsatisfactory overall score.

Work Documentation: Document findings in patient's chart.

Time Began ______________ Time Ended ______________

No.	Steps	Points	Check #1	Check #2	Check #3
1.	Use proper handwashing technique and apply PPE as appropriate before giving first aid.	10			
2.	Be calm and reassuring in approach to victim.	10			
3.	Do not thaw out the area unless it can be kept thawed.	10			
4.	Do not massage the area.	10			
5.	Do not use direct heat to thaw the area.	10			
6.	Remove any constricting clothes or jewelry.	10			
7.	To thaw the frozen area, place it in warm water or apply a warm cloth; keep water or cloth warm (not hot) until area softens and color and sensation return; as the area thaws, pain and swelling can be expected.	10			
8.	After thawing, apply a sterile, dry dressing.	10			
9.	If fingers or toes are frostbitten, place a dressing between them.	10			
10.	Move the thawed area as little as possible.	10			

© 2017 Cengage Learning. All Rights Reserved. May not be scanned, copied or duplicated, or posted to a publicly accessible website, in whole or in part.

No.	Steps	Points	Check #1	Check #2	Check #3
11.	Discourage smoking or drinking alcohol.	10			
	Student's Total Points				
	Points Possible	110			
	Final Score (Student's Total Points/ Possible Points)				

CHART FINDINGS

____

____

Instructor's/Evaluator's Comments and Suggestions:

____

____

____

____

Evaluator's Signature: ______________________ **Date:** ____________

© 2017 Cengage Learning. All Rights Reserved. May not be scanned, copied or duplicated, or posted to a publicly accessible website, in whole or in part.

Name: ______________________________ Date: __________ Score: __________

Procedure Assessment 21-8b: Temperature-Related Illnesses—Hypothermia

Task: Giving first aid for hypothermia

Standard: Complete the skill in 5 minutes with a minimum of 70% within three attempts.

Scoring: Divide points earned by total possible points. Failure to perform any of the following critical steps will result in an unsatisfactory overall score.

Work Documentation: Document findings in patient's chart.

Time Began ____________________ Time Ended ____________________

No.	Steps	Points	Check #1	Check #2	Check #3
1.	Use proper handwashing technique and apply PPE as appropriate before giving first aid.	10			
2.	Be calm and reassuring in approach to victim.	10			
3.	If frostbite and hypothermia are present, treat the hypothermia first.	10			
4.	If respirations are below 6 per minute, begin rescue breathing.	10			
5.	If possible, gently move the victim to a shelter.	10			
6.	Remove wet clothes and replace them with dry ones.	10			
7.	Remove constricting clothes and jewelry.	10			
8.	Do not use direct heat.	10			
9.	Apply warm packs (towels or linens) to the neck, chest, and groin.	10			
10.	If the victim is able to drink, give him or her warm, sweet fluids.	10			

© 2017 Cengage Learning. All Rights Reserved. May not be scanned, copied or duplicated, or posted to a publicly accessible website, in whole or in part.

No.	Steps	Points	Check #1	Check #2	Check #3
11.	Wrap the victim in a space blanket, or aluminum foil, including the neck and head; the rescuer can also place his or her own body next to the victim to warm him or her.	10			
	Student's Total Points				
	Points Possible	110			
	Final Score (Student's Total Points/ Possible Points)				

CHART FINDINGS

____

____

Instructor's/Evaluator's Comments and Suggestions:

____

____

____

____

Evaluator's Signature: ____________________ **Date:** ____________

© 2017 Cengage Learning. All Rights Reserved. May not be scanned, copied or duplicated, or posted to a publicly accessible website, in whole or in part.

Name: ______________________ Date: __________ Score: __________

Procedure Assessment 21-8c: Temperature-Related Illnesses—Heat Cramps

Task: Giving first aid for heat cramps

Standard: Complete the skill in 5 minutes with a minimum of 70% within three attempts.

Scoring: Divide points earned by total possible points. Failure to perform any of the following critical steps will result in an unsatisfactory overall score.

Work Documentation: Document findings in patient's chart.

Time Began ______________ Time Ended ______________

No.	Steps	Points	Check #1	Check #2	Check #3
1.	Use proper handwashing technique and apply PPE as appropriate before giving first aid.	10			
2.	Be calm and reassuring in approach to victim.	10			
3.	Do not give liquids that contain alcohol or caffeine.	10			
4.	Do not give any medication used to lower the temperature (e.g., aspirin or Tylenol).	10			
5.	Do not give salt tablets; instead use a salt-and-water solution or an electrolyte drink (e.g., Gatorade or Pedialyte).	10			
6.	Fan the victim.	10			
7.	Move the victim to the shade or a cooled room and elevate the feet if not prohibited (e.g., causes difficulty breathing; there's a head, neck, spine, or leg injury; or it makes the victim uncomfortable).	10			
8.	Apply cool water to the body (do not use alcohol rub); wrap the victim in cool towels and turn on fan.	10			
9.	Apply cold towels to the back of the neck, on the groin, and under the arms.	10			

© 2017 Cengage Learning. All Rights Reserved. May not be scanned, copied or duplicated, or posted to a publicly accessible website, in whole or in part.

No.	Steps	Points	Check #1	Check #2	Check #3
10.	When the temperature lowers to 100°F, the cooling effort can be stopped, but monitor victim closely for the next 2–4 hours.	10			
	Student's Total Points				
	Points Possible	100			
	Final Score (Student's Total Points/ Possible Points)				

CHART FINDINGS

____

____

Instructor's/Evaluator's Comments and Suggestions:

____

____

____

____

Evaluator's Signature: ______________________ **Date:** ____________

© 2017 Cengage Learning. All Rights Reserved. May not be scanned, copied or duplicated, or posted to a publicly accessible website, in whole or in part.

Name: ______________________ Date: __________ Score: __________

Procedure Assessment 21-8d: Temperature-Related Illnesses—Heat Stroke

Task: Giving first aid for heat stroke

Standard: Complete the skill in 3 minutes with a minimum of 70% within three attempts.

Scoring: Divide points earned by total possible points. Failure to perform any of the following critical steps will result in an unsatisfactory overall score.

Work Documentation: Document findings in patient's chart.

Time Began ____________ Time Ended ____________

No.	Steps	Points	Check #1	Check #2	Check #3
1.	Use proper handwashing technique and apply PPE as appropriate before giving first aid.	10			
2.	Be calm and reassuring in approach to victim.	10			
3.	Call EMS.	10			
4.	Do not give liquids to a victim with heat stroke.	10			
5.	If EMS is not immediately available, immerse victim in cold water, but monitor his or her alertness, pulse, and respirations closely.	10			
	Student's Total Points				
	Points Possible	50			
	Final Score (Student's Total Points/ Possible Points)				

CHART FINDINGS

____

____

Instructor's/Evaluator's Comments and Suggestions:

____

____

____

____

Evaluator's Signature: ______________________ **Date:** ____________

© 2017 Cengage Learning. All Rights Reserved. May not be scanned, copied or duplicated, or posted to a publicly accessible website, in whole or in part.

Name: ______________________ Date: __________ Score: __________

Procedure Assessment 21-9a: Common Conditions—Breathing Difficulty

Task: Giving first aid for breathing difficulty

Standard: Complete the skill in 5 minutes with a minimum of 70% within three attempts.

Scoring: Divide points earned by total possible points. Failure to perform any of the following critical steps will result in an unsatisfactory overall score.

Work Documentation: Document findings in patient's chart.

Time Began ____________ Time Ended ____________

No.	Steps	Points	Check #1	Check #2	Check #3
1.	Use proper handwashing technique and apply PPE as appropriate before giving first aid.	10			
2.	Be calm and reassuring in approach to victim.	10			
3.	Do not place a pillow under the victim's head.	10			
4.	Loosen any constricting clothing and assist the victim into the most comfortable position, unless neck or back injury is suspected.	10			
5.	Ask the victim if there is any medication he or she takes for the problem (e.g., an asthmatic may have an inhaler with them).	10			
6.	Call EMS and keep the victim safe and comfortable until help arrives.	10			
	Student's Total Points				
	Points Possible	60			
	Final Score (Student's Total Points/ Possible Points)				

© 2017 Cengage Learning. All Rights Reserved. May not be scanned, copied or duplicated, or posted to a publicly accessible website, in whole or in part.

CHART FINDINGS

____

____

Instructor's/Evaluator's Comments and Suggestions:

____

____

____

____

Evaluator's Signature: ______________________________ **Date:** ________________

© 2017 Cengage Learning. All Rights Reserved. May not be scanned, copied or duplicated, or posted to a publicly accessible website, in whole or in part.

Name: ______________________ Date: __________ Score: __________

Procedure Assessment 21-9b: Common Conditions—Hyperventilation

Task: Giving first aid for hyperventilation

Standard: Complete the skill in 3 minutes with a minimum of 70% within three attempts.

Scoring: Divide points earned by total possible points. Failure to perform any of the following critical steps will result in an unsatisfactory overall score.

Work Documentation: Document findings in patient's chart.

Time Began ______________ Time Ended ______________

No.	Steps	Points	Check #1	Check #2	Check #3
1.	Use proper handwashing technique and apply PPE as appropriate before giving first aid.	10			
2.	Be calm and reassuring in approach to victim.	10			
3.	Victims should breathe into a paper bag, hold one nostril closed (make sure the mouth is closed) while breathing, or have them cup their hands over their mouth and nose while breathing.	10			
4.	Encouraging the victim to talk is often helpful.	10			
	Student's Total Points				
	Points Possible	40			
	Final Score (Student's Total Points/ Possible Points)				

CHART FINDINGS

____

____

Instructor's/Evaluator's Comments and Suggestions:

____

____

____

____

Evaluator's Signature: ______________________ **Date:** ______________

© 2017 Cengage Learning. All Rights Reserved. May not be scanned, copied or duplicated, or posted to a publicly accessible website, in whole or in part.

Name: ______________________ Date: __________ Score: __________

Procedure Assessment 21-9c: Common Conditions—Chest Pain (Angina)

Task: Giving first aid for chest pain (angina)

Standard: Complete the skill in 5 minutes with a minimum of 70% within three attempts.

Scoring: Divide points earned by total possible points. Failure to perform any of the following critical steps will result in an unsatisfactory overall score.

Work Documentation: Document findings in patient's chart.

Time Began ______________ Time Ended ______________

No.	Steps	Points	Check #1	Check #2	Check #3
1.	Use proper handwashing technique and apply PPE as appropriate before giving first aid.	10			
2.	Be calm and reassuring in approach to victim.	10			
3.	Always call EMS immediately.	10			
4.	Have the victim stop any activity he or she was doing.	10			
5.	If the victim has medication for angina, assist him or her in taking it.	10			
6.	Do not give the victim anything to eat or drink.	10			
7.	Loosen any constricting clothing and keep the victim warm.	10			
8.	Stay with the victim until help arrives.	10			
9.	Start rescue breathing if he or she stops breathing, or give full CPR if the heart stops.	10			
	Student's Total Points				
	Points Possible	90			
	Final Score (Student's Total Points/ Possible Points)				

© 2017 Cengage Learning. All Rights Reserved. May not be scanned, copied or duplicated, or posted to a publicly accessible website, in whole or in part.

CHART FINDINGS

____

____

Instructor's/Evaluator's Comments and Suggestions:

____

____

____

____

Evaluator's Signature: ______________________ **Date:** ____________

© 2017 Cengage Learning. All Rights Reserved. May not be scanned, copied or duplicated, or posted to a publicly accessible website, in whole or in part.

Name: ______________________ Date: __________ Score: __________

Procedure Assessment 21-9d: Common Conditions—Diabetes

Task: Giving first aid for diabetes

Standard: Complete the skill in 5 minutes with a minimum of 70% within three attempts.

Scoring: Divide points earned by total possible points. Failure to perform any of the following critical steps will result in an unsatisfactory overall score.

Work Documentation: Document findings in patient's chart.

Time Began __________________ Time Ended __________________

No.	Steps	Points	Check #1	Check #2	Check #3
1.	Use proper handwashing technique and apply PPE as appropriate before giving first aid.	10			
2.	Be calm and reassuring in approach to victim.	10			
3.	If the victim states that his or her blood sugar is too high and he or she needs to have an insulin injection, assist the victim with the administration of the medication.	10			
4.	Get medical help and stay with the victim to monitor his or her condition.	10			
5.	If the victim is conscious, give him or her unsweetened liquids.	10			
6.	If the victim states that his or her blood sugar is too low, immediately give something sweet (e.g., fruit juice, sugar in water, candy). If this is the problem, the victim should improve within 5–15 minutes after administration of the sweet.	10			
7.	When recovered, the victim should eat some protein and carbohydrates (e.g., crackers and cheese or peanut butter and bread).	10			
8.	If the victim does not recover or is unconscious, call EMS.	10			

© 2017 Cengage Learning. All Rights Reserved. May not be scanned, copied or duplicated, or posted to a publicly accessible website, in whole or in part.

No.	Steps	Points	Check #1	Check #2	Check #3
9.	If in doubt as to whether it is high or low blood sugar, treat it with something sweet.	10			
	Student's Total Points				
	Points Possible	90			
	Final Score (Student's Total Points/ Possible Points)				

CHART FINDINGS

____

____

Instructor's/Evaluator's Comments and Suggestions:

____

____

____

____

Evaluator's Signature: ______________________________ **Date:** ______________

© 2017 Cengage Learning. All Rights Reserved. May not be scanned, copied or duplicated, or posted to a publicly accessible website, in whole or in part.

Name: ______________________ Date: __________ Score: __________

Procedure Assessment 21-9e: Common Conditions—Fainting (Syncope)

Task: Giving first aid for fainting (syncope)

Standard: Complete the skill in 5 minutes with a minimum of 70% within three attempts.

Scoring: Divide points earned by total possible points. Failure to perform any of the following critical steps will result in an unsatisfactory overall score.

Work Documentation: Document findings in patient's chart.

Time Began ______________ Time Ended ______________

No.	Steps	Points	Check #1	Check #2	Check #3
1.	Use proper handwashing technique and apply PPE as appropriate before giving first aid.	10			
2.	Be calm and reassuring in approach to victim.	10			
3.	If you're present when victim is falling, assist him or her gently to the floor.	10			
4.	Place the victim on his or her back and elevate the legs 8–12 inches.	10			
5.	Do not place a pillow under the head.	10			
6.	Loosen any constricting clothing.	10			
7.	Do not attempt to awaken the victim by throwing water on him or her, shaking, or slapping the face.	10			
8.	If vomiting occurs turn the head to the side.	10			
9.	Call EMS if the victim is not alert within approximately 5 minutes, is elderly, or other signs and symptoms are noted that may indicate another problem.	10			
	Student's Total Points				
	Points Possible	90			
	Final Score (Student's Total Points/ Possible Points)				

© 2017 Cengage Learning. All Rights Reserved. May not be scanned, copied or duplicated, or posted to a publicly accessible website, in whole or in part.

CHART FINDINGS

Instructor's/Evaluator's Comments and Suggestions:

Evaluator's Signature: ________________ **Date:** ________________

© 2017 Cengage Learning. All Rights Reserved. May not be scanned, copied or duplicated, or posted to a publicly accessible website, in whole or in part.

Name: ______________________ Date: ________ Score: ________

Procedure Assessment 21-9f: Common Conditions—Hyperthermia

Task: Giving first aid for fever (hyperthermia)

Standard: Complete the skill in 5 minutes with a minimum of 70% within three attempts.

Scoring: Divide points earned by total possible points. Failure to perform any of the following critical steps will result in an unsatisfactory overall score.

Work Documentation: Document findings in patient's chart.

Time Began ______________ Time Ended ______________

No.	Steps	Points	Check #1	Check #2	Check #3
1.	Use proper handwashing technique and apply PPE as appropriate before giving first aid.	10			
2.	Be calm and reassuring in approach to victim.	10			
3.	Remove excess clothing and blankets.	10			
4.	Gently cool the victim by sponging him or her with lukewarm water.	10			
5.	Call the physician at once for further instructions, such as giving medication to bring the fever down (e.g., aspirin or Tylenol).	10			
6.	Even lower fevers that persist over 24 hours need to be evaluated.	10			
7.	Call EMS if victim is having difficulty breathing, has unusual skin color, a stiff neck, or appears ill.	10			
	Student's Total Points				
	Points Possible	70			
	Final Score (Student's Total Points/ Possible Points)				

© 2017 Cengage Learning. All Rights Reserved. May not be scanned, copied or duplicated, or posted to a publicly accessible website, in whole or in part.

CHART FINDINGS

____

____

Instructor's/Evaluator's Comments and Suggestions:

____

____

____

____

Evaluator's Signature: ______________________ **Date:** ____________

© 2017 Cengage Learning. All Rights Reserved. May not be scanned, copied or duplicated, or posted to a publicly accessible website, in whole or in part.

Name: ________________________ Date: __________ Score: __________

Procedure Assessment 21-9g: Common Conditions—Drowning

Task: Giving first aid for drowning

Standard: Complete the skill in 5 minutes with a minimum of 70% within three attempts.

Scoring: Divide points earned by total possible points. Failure to perform any of the following critical steps will result in an unsatisfactory overall score.

Work Documentation: Document findings in patient's chart.

Time Began ________________ Time Ended ________________

No.	Steps	Points	Check #1	Check #2	Check #3
1.	Use proper handwashing technique and apply PPE as appropriate before giving first aid.	10			
2.	Be calm and reassuring in approach to victim.	10			
3.	Be on the alert for irregular swimming strokes, when only the head is above the water, and if the person is fully dressed.	10			
4.	Call EMS.	10			
5.	Rescue the drowning victim if you can do so without endangering yourself. It is best not to enter the water, but to extend a stick, life preserver, or some other object for the victim to grab and then pull him or her to safety.	10			
6.	Do rescue breathing and treat the victim for hypothermia as needed. Do full CPR if no pulse is present.	10			
	Student's Total Points				
	Points Possible	60			
	Final Score (Student's Total Points/ Possible Points)				

© 2017 Cengage Learning. All Rights Reserved. May not be scanned, copied or duplicated, or posted to a publicly accessible website, in whole or in part.

CHART FINDINGS

____

____

Instructor's/Evaluator's Comments and Suggestions:

____

____

____

____

Evaluator's Signature: ________________________________ **Date:** __________________

© 2017 Cengage Learning. All Rights Reserved. May not be scanned, copied or duplicated, or posted to a publicly accessible website, in whole or in part.

Name: ______________________ Date: __________ Score: __________

Procedure Assessment 21-9h: Common Conditions—Seizures (Convulsions)

Task: Giving first aid for seizures (convulsions)

Standard: Complete the skill in 5 minutes with a minimum of 70% within three attempts.

Scoring: Divide points earned by total possible points. Failure to perform any of the following critical steps will result in an unsatisfactory overall score.

Work Documentation: Document findings in patient's chart.

Time Began ______________ Time Ended ______________

No.	Steps	Points	Check #1	Check #2	Check #3
1.	Use proper handwashing technique and apply PPE as appropriate before giving first aid.	10			
2.	Be calm and reassuring in approach to victim.	10			
3.	If the victim is falling, support the victim as he or she falls.	10			
4.	Remove any sharp objects in the area.	10			
5.	Loosen tight clothing.	10			
6.	Do not place anything into the mouth, try to restrain the victim, move the victim (unless in danger), or perform rescue breathing during a seizure.	10			
7.	Do not try to keep the victim awake, but place him or her on the stomach or side (if you suspect neck or back injury, roll the body as a unit to a side-lying position, while keeping the spine in straight alignment). Protect the airway if vomiting occurs.	10			
8.	Call EMS.	10			
	Student's Total Points				
	Points Possible	80			
	Final Score (Student's Total Points/ Possible Points)				

© 2017 Cengage Learning. All Rights Reserved. May not be scanned, copied or duplicated, or posted to a publicly accessible website, in whole or in part.

CHART FINDINGS

____

____

Instructor's/Evaluator's Comments and Suggestions:

____

____

____

____

Evaluator's Signature: ______________________ **Date:** ______________

© 2017 Cengage Learning. All Rights Reserved. May not be scanned, copied or duplicated, or posted to a publicly accessible website, in whole or in part.

Name: ______________________ Date: __________ Score: __________

Procedure Assessment 21-9i: Common Conditions—Shock

Task: Giving first aid for shock

Standard: Complete the skill in 5 minutes with a minimum of 70% within three attempts.

Scoring: Divide points earned by total possible points. Failure to perform any of the following critical steps will result in an unsatisfactory overall score.

Work Documentation: Document findings in patient's chart.

Time Began ______________ Time Ended ______________

No.	Steps	Points	Check #1	Check #2	Check #3
1.	Use proper handwashing technique and apply PPE as appropriate before giving first aid.	10			
2.	Be calm and reassuring in approach to victim.	10			
3.	Call EMS.	10			
4.	Place the victim in the shock position if there is no neck or back injury.	10			
5.	Turn the victim's head to the side if there is vomiting or drooling.	10			
6.	Do not elevate the head.	10			
7.	Loosen restricting clothes and keep the victim warm.	10			
8.	Do not give the victim any liquids or food.	10			
9.	Give first aid for any underlying illness or injury.	10			
10.	Do not use the shock position if it is uncomfortable.	10			
11.	Do not use the shock position if the victim has a sting or bite in the lower limbs.	10			
12.	Stay with the victim and assist as needed until medical help arrives.	10			
	Student's Total Points				
	Points Possible	120			
	Final Score (Student's Total Points/ Possible Points)				

© 2017 Cengage Learning. All Rights Reserved. May not be scanned, copied or duplicated, or posted to a publicly accessible website, in whole or in part.

CHART FINDINGS

____

____

Instructor's/Evaluator's Comments and Suggestions:

____

____

____

____

Evaluator's Signature: ______________________ **Date:** ____________

© 2017 Cengage Learning. All Rights Reserved. May not be scanned, copied or duplicated, or posted to a publicly accessible website, in whole or in part.

Name: ______________________ Date: __________ Score: __________

Procedure Assessment 21-9j: Common Conditions—Stroke or Cerebrovascular Accident (CVA)

Task: Giving first aid for stroke or cerebrovascular accident (CVA)

Standard: Complete the skill in 3 minutes with a minimum of 70% within three attempts.

Scoring: Divide points earned by total possible points. Failure to perform any of the following critical steps will result in an unsatisfactory overall score.

Work Documentation: Document findings in patient's chart.

Time Began ______________ Time Ended ______________

No.	Steps	Points	Check #1	Check #2	Check #3
1.	Use proper handwashing technique and apply PPE as appropriate before giving first aid.	10			
2.	Be calm and reassuring in approach to victim.	10			
3.	Call EMS.	10			
4.	Help the victim get into a comfortable position.	10			
5.	Give no liquids or food by mouth.	10			
6.	Stay with the victim and assist as needed until medical help arrives.	10			
	Student's Total Points				
	Points Possible	60			
	Final Score (Student's Total Points/ Possible Points)				

CHART FINDINGS

____

____

Instructor's/Evaluator's Comments and Suggestions:

____

____

____

____

Evaluator's Signature: ______________________ **Date:** ______________

© 2017 Cengage Learning. All Rights Reserved. May not be scanned, copied or duplicated, or posted to a publicly accessible website, in whole or in part.

Name: ______________________ Date: __________ Score: __________

Procedure Assessment 21-9k: Common Conditions—Unconsciousness

Task: Giving first aid for unconsciousness

Standard: Complete the skill in 5 minutes with a minimum of 70% within three attempts.

Scoring: Divide points earned by total possible points. Failure to perform any of the following critical steps will result in an unsatisfactory overall score.

Work Documentation: Document findings in patient's chart.

Time Began ______________ Time Ended ______________

No.	Steps	Points	Check #1	Check #2	Check #3
1.	Use proper handwashing technique and apply PPE as appropriate before giving first aid.	10			
2.	Be calm and reassuring in approach to victim.	10			
3.	Call EMS if the victim does not quickly regain consciousness (i.e., faints) or if illness or injury is evident.	10			
4.	The goal of the treatment of the unconscious victim is to maintain the airway.	10			
5.	Do not give anything by mouth.	10			
6.	Keep the victim warm.	10			
7.	If there is no neck or back injury, place the victim in the recovery position by turning the head to the side, or turn the entire body to the side or onto the abdomen.	10			
8.	Gently tilt the victim's head back.	10			
9.	If neck or back injury is suspected, leave the victim in the position in which you find him or her unless the victim is having difficulty breathing. If there is difficulty in breathing, choking, or vomiting, roll the entire body as a unit to a side-lying position while keeping the spine in straight alignment.	10			

© 2017 Cengage Learning. All Rights Reserved. May not be scanned, copied or duplicated, or posted to a publicly accessible website, in whole or in part.

No.	Steps	Points	Check #1	Check #2	Check #3
10.	Enlist the assistance of bystanders, if possible, when moving the victim to ensure the head, neck, and back stay in a straight line.	10			
11.	Give first aid for any underlying illness or injury.	10			
12.	If the victim becomes restless, you may have to gently restrain him or her.	10			
13.	Stay with the victim until medical assistance arrives.	10			
	Student's Total Points				
	Points Possible	130			
	Final Score (Student's Total Points/ Possible Points)				

CHART FINDINGS

____

____

Instructor's/Evaluator's Comments and Suggestions:

____

____

____

____

Evaluator's Signature: ______________________ **Date:** ____________

© 2017 Cengage Learning. All Rights Reserved. May not be scanned, copied or duplicated, or posted to a publicly accessible website, in whole or in part.

Name: ______________________ Date: __________ Score: __________

Procedure Assessment 21-10: Triangular Sling

Task: Applying a triangular sling

Standard: Complete the skill in 5 minutes with a minimum of 70% within three attempts.

Scoring: Divide points earned by total possible points. Failure to perform any of the following critical steps will result in an unsatisfactory overall score.

Work Documentation: Document findings in patient's chart.

Time Began ____________________ Time Ended ____________________

No.	Steps	Points	Check #1	Check #2	Check #3
1.	Use proper handwashing technique before applying a sling.	10			
2.	Support the injured part and slide the sling under the arm on the victim's injured side.	10			
3.	Place top corner over the victim's noninjured shoulder.	10			
4.	Pull the bottom corner of the sling up past the victim's chin and over the shoulder on the injured side. Leave the fingers showing.	10			
5.	Tie the sling around the victim's neck, placing it a little to one side.	10			
6.	Fold over the extra cloth at the victim's elbow and secure it with a safety pin. Place your hand between the bandage and the victim's skin when inserting a pin.	10			
7.	Check for circulation.	10			
	Student's Total Points				
	Points Possible	70			
	Final Score (Student's Total Points/ Possible Points)				

© 2017 Cengage Learning. All Rights Reserved. May not be scanned, copied or duplicated, or posted to a publicly accessible website, in whole or in part.

CHART FINDINGS

____

____

Instructor's/Evaluator's Comments and Suggestions:

____

____

____

____

Evaluator's Signature: ______________________________ **Date:** ______________

© 2017 Cengage Learning. All Rights Reserved. May not be scanned, copied or duplicated, or posted to a publicly accessible website, in whole or in part.

Name: ______________________ Date: __________ Score: __________

Procedure Assessment 21-11: Spiral Wrap

Task: Applying a spiral wrap bandage

Standard: Complete the skill in 5 minutes with a minimum of 70% within three attempts.

Scoring: Divide points earned by total possible points. Failure to perform any of the following critical steps will result in an unsatisfactory overall score.

Work Documentation: Document findings in patient's chart.

Time Began ______________ Time Ended ______________

No.	Steps	Points	Check #1	Check #2	Check #3
1.	Use proper handwashing technique before applying a bandage.	10			
2.	Start wrap at distal end.	10			
3.	Anchor the bandage by leaving a corner exposed. The corner is then folded down and covered when the bandage is circled around the limb.	10			
4.	Overlap each rotation over the previous one by approximately half of the wrap.	10			
5.	Place your hand between the bandage and the victim's skin if inserting a pin; can also secure with tape.	10			
6.	Verify circulation in the fingers and toes if it's used on the arm or leg.	10			
7.	Verify ease of breathing if wrap is on the trunk.	10			
	Student's Total Points				
	Points Possible	70			
	Final Score (Student's Total Points/ Possible Points)				

© 2017 Cengage Learning. All Rights Reserved. May not be scanned, copied or duplicated, or posted to a publicly accessible website, in whole or in part.

CHART FINDINGS

____

____

Instructor's/Evaluator's Comments and Suggestions:

____

____

____

____

Evaluator's Signature: ______________________________ **Date:** ______________

© 2017 Cengage Learning. All Rights Reserved. May not be scanned, copied or duplicated, or posted to a publicly accessible website, in whole or in part.

Name: ______________________ Date: __________ Score: __________

Procedure Assessment 21-12: Figure-Eight Wrap

Task: Applying a figure-eight wrap bandage

Standard: Complete the skill in 5 minutes with a minimum of 70% within three attempts.

Scoring: Divide points earned by total possible points. Failure to perform any of the following critical steps will result in an unsatisfactory overall score.

Work Documentation: Document findings in patient's chart.

Time Began ______________ Time Ended ______________

No.	Steps	Points	Check #1	Check #2	Check #3
1.	Use proper handwashing technique before applying a bandage.	10			
2.	Anchor the bandage at the instep and wrap several times around the instep. Then bring the wrap up diagonally over the foot.	10			
3.	Bring the bandage around back of the ankle and then down over the top of the foot and back under the instep.	10			
4.	Repeat the figure-eight pattern, moving the wrap out in both directions (up the leg and toward the toes) with each repeat of the pattern while overlapping approximately half of the previous layer.	10			
5.	When completed, wrap around the ankle several times and secure the end.	10			
6.	Check circulation distal to the wrap.	10			
	Student's Total Points				
	Points Possible	60			
	Final Score (Student's Total Points/ Possible Points)				

© 2017 Cengage Learning. All Rights Reserved. May not be scanned, copied or duplicated, or posted to a publicly accessible website, in whole or in part.

CHART FINDINGS

____

____

Instructor's/Evaluator's Comments and Suggestions:

____

____

____

____

Evaluator's Signature: ______________________ **Date:** ____________

© 2017 Cengage Learning. All Rights Reserved. May not be scanned, copied or duplicated, or posted to a publicly accessible website, in whole or in part.

Name: ______________________ Date: __________ Score: __________

Procedure Assessment 21-13: Finger Bandage

Task: Applying a bandage to a finger

Standard: Complete the skill in 5 minutes with a minimum of 70% within three attempts.

Scoring: Divide points earned by total possible points. Failure to perform any of the following critical steps will result in an unsatisfactory overall score.

Work Documentation: Document findings in patient's chart.

Time Began ______________ Time Ended ______________

No.	Steps	Points	Check #1	Check #2	Check #3
1.	Use proper handwashing technique before applying a bandage.	10			
2.	Place the end of the wrap at the bottom of one side of the finger and fold it over the tip of the finger and down to the bottom of the other side of the finger. Repeat this three to four times.	10			
3.	Start at the bottom of the finger and spiral the wrap up and down finger	10			
4.	Secure by doing several figure-eight wraps around the wrist.	10			
5.	When the figure-eight wrap is complete, circle the wrist several times. Split the wrap and tie in a knot.	10			
6.	Monitor patient. If any signs of decreased circulation occur, loosen the wrap immediately.	10			
	Student's Total Points				
	Points Possible	60			
	Final Score (Student's Total Points/ Possible Points)				

© 2017 Cengage Learning. All Rights Reserved. May not be scanned, copied or duplicated, or posted to a publicly accessible website, in whole or in part.

CHART FINDINGS

____

____

Instructor's/Evaluator's Comments and Suggestions:

____

____

____

____

Evaluator's Signature: ______________________________ **Date:** ______________

© 2017 Cengage Learning. All Rights Reserved. May not be scanned, copied or duplicated, or posted to a publicly accessible website, in whole or in part.